A Beacon of Under...
When Sense and Sanity ...

Are you tired of reading about others' experiences with Kundalini and the chakras? Or sick of the intellectual sleight-of-hand by which charlatans have bandied about these concepts without regard for what is really active and changing within your system? Whenever you feel as though you are operating a few cylinders short, you are accessing only a portion of your available Kundalini energy.

It is our birthright to evolve, develop, and become super-people. Life's simplest problems may have imbalanced or blocked Kundalini flow at their root. Everyone has Kundalini, just as everyone has sexual impulses. In light of today's tenor of cosmic flux, not to know about Kundalini is tantamount to refusing teenagers sex education. The more we know, the more choices we have.

Whether you have experienced the "big release" spontaneously but have been ill-equipped to channel its force in a productive manner, or whether your Kundalini is dormant like a wintering bear but poised to wake up ravenous for knowledge in the Spring of a new personal consciousness, this book is your guide to satiating the strange, new appetites which result when life-in-process "blows open" your body's many energy centers.

As the energies of the Aquarian Age intensify, more and more people are horrified, frightened or even incapacitated by indescribably powerful spontaneous Kundalini releases. In many cases, people have no idea what's happening to them, and, reacting with ignorance to symptoms of illness or insanity, worsen what already seems like an impossible situation.

For the newcomer to Kundalini and the chakras, this book is a blessing. It provides detailed instructions for initiating preliminary system-cleansing in preparation for release. Because Kundalini energy is sometimes so potent that its "human module" finds it difficult to function in daily routine and commitments, the author provides methods for moderating or holding its release in check.

With personal-scale evolution suddenly on a strident quantum-track, there is a great need for guidance to soften transitions between our various states of being in our process of evolution. Knowing and understanding Kundalini does make the process much easier on body, mind, and spirit.

About the Author

Genevieve Lewis Paulson is the director and owner of Dimensions of Evolvement, located on 165 acres of the Ozark mountains in Arkansas, a center of psychic, personal and spiritual learning, accrediting students in the study of Kundalini energy development.

Not your typical "new ager," Ms. Paulson is steeped in Western Christian tradition and once served as administrator of a United Methodist Church. With the onset of a fierce Kundalini upsurge in 1968 she began her profound energy arousal, sought accreditation as a group leader in the fields of sensitivity training and conflict management—still under the purview of the Church—only later discovering the ancient literature to describe the Kundalini awakening she had been undergoing. In the early 1970s she founded Sunergos, Inc., a spiritual growth center in Chicago. Where her new experiences might have led her to abandon Western religious beliefs, she instead found a method to meld two varieties of truth, creating a synthesis of two great traditions of belief.

At present not content simply to sip herbal tea and watch the turkey buzzards circle over the Ozarks, Genevieve lives like an itinerant preacher in her second home, a red pickup truck, counseling and giving workshops throughout the year on a circuit of cities from Florida to Arizona.

To Write to the Author

If you wish to contact the author or would like more information about this book, please write to the author in care of Llewellyn Worldwide and we will forward your request. Both the author and publisher appreciate hearing from you and learning of your enjoyment of this book and how it has helped you. Llewellyn Worldwide cannot guarantee that every letter written to the author can be answered, but all will be forwarded. Please write to:

Genevieve Lewis Paulson
c/o Llewellyn Worldwide
P.O. Box 64383-592, St. Paul, MN 55164-0383, U.S.A.

Please enclose a self-addressed, stamped envelope for reply, or $1.00 to cover costs. If outside the U.S.A., enclose international postal reply coupon.

Free Catalog from Llewellyn

For more than 90 years Llewellyn has brought its readers knowledge in the fields of metaphysics and human potential. Learn about the newest books in spiritual guidance, natural healing, astrology, occult philosophy and more. Enjoy book reviews, new age articles, a calendar of events, plus current advertised products and services. To get your free copy of *Llewellyn's New Worlds of Mind and Spirit*, send your name and address to:

Llewellyn's New Worlds of Mind and Spirit
P.O. Box 64383-592, St. Paul, MN 55164-0383, U.S.A.

Llewellyn's New Age Series

Kundalini and the Chakras

A Practical Manual—Evolution in This Lifetime

Genevieve Lewis Paulson

1994
Llewellyn Publications
St. Paul, Minnesota 55164-0383, U.S.A.

FIRST EDITION
Fifth Printing, 1994

Cover Painting by Randy Asplund-Faith
Interior paintings and illustrations by Randy Asplund-Faith

Library of Congress Cataloging-in-Publication Data
    Paulson, Genevieve Lewis, 1927–
      Kundalini and the chakras : a practical manual—evolution in
    this lifetime / Genevieve Lewis Paulson.—1st ed.
    (Llewellyn's new age series)
      p.   cm.
    ISBN 0-87542-592-5
    1. Kundalini. 2. Chakras 3. Occultism. I. Title.
BL1238.56.K86P38   1991
  294.5'43—dc20   90-27422
                                                                         CIP

Llewellyn Publications
A Division of Llewellyn Worldwide, Ltd.
P.O. Box 64383, St. Paul, MN 55164-0383

About Llewellyn's New Age Series

The "New Age"—it's a phrase we use, but what does it mean? Does it mean that we are entering the Aquarian Age? Does it mean that a new Messiah is coming to correct all that is wrong and make Earth into a Garden? Probably not—but the idea of a *major change* is there, combined with awareness that Earth *can* be a Garden; that war, crime, poverty, disease, etc., are not necessary "evils."

Optimists, dreamers, scientists ... nearly all of us believe in a "better tomorrow," and that somehow we can do things now that will make for a better future life for ourselves and for coming generations.

In one sense, we all know there's nothing new under the Heavens, and in another sense that every day makes a new world. The difference is in our consciousness. And this is what the New Age is all about: it's a major change in consciousness found within each of us as we learn to bring forth and manifest powers that humanity has always potentially had.

Evolution moves in "leaps." Individuals struggle to develop talents and powers, and their efforts build a "power bank" in the Collective Unconsciousness, the soul of humanity that suddenly makes these same talents and powers easier access for the majority.

You still have to learn the "rules" for developing and applying these powers, but it is more like a "re-learning" than a *new* learning, because with the New Age it is as if the basis for these had become genetic.

Other Publications by the Author

Meditation and Human Growth

(The following books are not available from Llewellyn—contact the author for information:)

The Seven Bodies of Man in the Evolution of Consciousness
The Seven Eyes in the Evolution of Consciousness
Introduction to Basic Meditation
Use of Color and White Light
Introduction to Out of Body Travel
Quick Fixes
Prayer is an Altered State

Dedication

This book is dedicated to all my Kundalini students, but especially to the advanced group, who call themselves the "Indy-Yucky" group (Indiana and Kentucky); their willingness and enthusiasm have always delighted me. I also dedicate this book to my children; Stephen, Kari, Nina, Bradley, and Roger.

Appreciation

Special thanks to Ralph Thiel, who not only put the entire manuscript on computer, through many revisions, but helped with editing as well.

Special thanks also to Helen McMahan for the "Chakra Meditation" that appears in this book and for all her other help.

To Dave and Jo Bahn, who helped in so many ways.

To Richard Gilbert, for compiling the chart on the Chakras of the Seven Bodies and Planes.

Thanks also to Jim Blackfeather, Marge Schulz, Ruth Allen, Aaron Parker, Janet Irwin, Alice Shewmaker, Luanne Thiel, and Julie Thiel, Anne Lindstrom, and Nina Paulson.

My appreciation also goes to those whose interest and support were so helpful: son Stephen, daughter-in-law RaeJean, Joe Stamper, Gene Kieffer, Car and Jewell Foster.

TABLE OF CONTENTS

Foreword

Kundalini was a totally unknown word to me when I first became aware of its power. It was some time before I realized what had happened. I did have the help of direct guidance through clairaudience from Beings who guided me through the various stages. Much of the information in this book came to me originally from these Beings.

When I became aware of what was going on, I began the frantic search for any books which could give me corroboration concerning the information I was receiving! Such information was very scarce in the 1960s; I was grateful for anything I could find. Other verification came through my work with students.

It was not an easy road (the worst of it took seven years); it was interesting, traumatic sometimes, enlightening other times—but not easy. I came from a traditional church background, even serving as administrator of a 700-plus congregation at one time; opening up to these new concepts was strange. Later, my understanding of Christianity was strengthened through what I was learning. Kundalini certainly is a basis for religious and belief systems.

Kundalini is not exactly a household word yet, but increasing numbers of people are not only aware of it but living with its experiences. The "Kundalini Blues" are not yet an acceptable reason for staying home from work or not keeping up your end of things; I hope this book will help you not only keep up with your life but bring optimum evolutionary change into it.

Even though I had guidance from the Beings, and a lot of faith and help from others, the journey was still lonely. So are all spiritual journeys. Get yourself a journal to talk to. It always listens, never interrupts, and remembers what you write. Another reason for keeping a record of your experiences is that you, too, may write a book about Kundalini someday.

I hope this book will alleviate some of the concerns, questions, and loneliness you may have. I wouldn't trade the journey I've had and still have for anything. May you find it worth your while as well.

—Genevieve Lewis Paulson
Melbourne, Arkansas

Chapter 1

Kundalini: the Evolutionary Energy

Introduction

Everyone has an inner drive to excel or be special at something—to be unique. Sometimes people reach for this in negative ways. The underlying drive in all people, however, is one of evolution—to reach for enlightenment, to be God-like while still human.

In the Upanishads, it is expressed:

> Dwelling in this very body, we have somehow realized Brahman [expansion, evolution, the Absolute, Creator, Preserver, and Destroyer of the universe]; otherwise we should have remained ignorant and great destruction would have overtaken us. Those who know Brahman become immortal while others only suffer misery. [IV, iv, 14/Swami Nikhilananda translation.]

In the New Testament, Jesus answered:

> Is it not written in your own law, "I said: You are gods"? Those who are called gods to whom the word of God was delivered— and Scripture can not be set aside." [John 10:34-35/The New English Bible][1]

We find that we are all called to go beyond our humanness toward greater heights. The Kundalini energy pushes each of us toward this goal of enlightenment—knowing the light, knowing God.

---

1. "This is my sentence: Gods you may be, sons all of you of a high god,..." [Psalm 82:6]

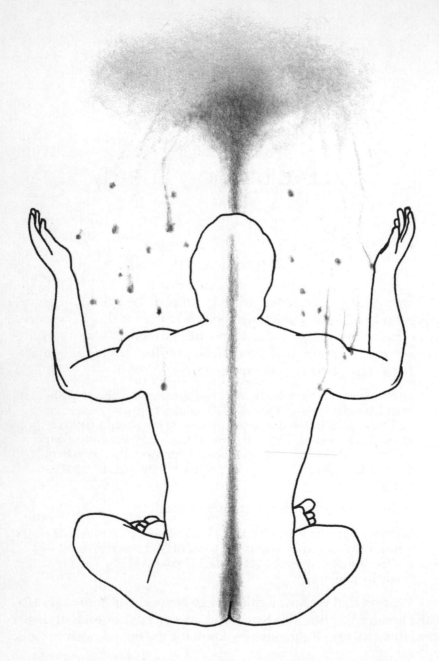

The red-orange of the Kundalini rises up the spine and mixes with divine energy (union of Shakti and Shakta). The colors turn golden, or sometimes silver.

In Tibetan Yoga and in other secret doctrines, it is expressed:

> By means of Shakti Yoga [energy discipline], the Tantric yogin attains discipline of body and mind and then proceeds to the mighty task of awakening the dormant, or innate, powers of divinity within himself, personified as the sleeping Goddess Kundalini. ... Then, from the mystic union of Shakta [at the top of the head] and the Shakti, is born Enlightenment; and the Yogin has attained the Goal.[2]

Kundalini, a Sanskrit word meaning "circular power," is an individual's basic evolutionary force. Each of us is born with some of this energy already flowing. The amount available and usable determines whether a person has low intelligence, is a genius, or is somewhere in the middle.

It is not just a matter of using what we already have, but of awakening the much greater amount waiting in the Kundalini reservoir located at the base of the spine.

Kundalini is a natural force common to all of us. It is not a religion, although it is practiced by some religions and the process can enhance and develop each person's own religious beliefs.

Ancient Eastern literature contains a great deal of information on the Kundalini. This is not true of Western literature; but more is being written. As interest in the Aquarian Age grows rapidly and brings stronger energies to facilitate spontaneous Kundalini release, people in all walks of life, all ages and all levels of growth, experience Kundalini, regardless of cultural, philosophical or religious backgrounds.

Little information is available for people who have not even heard of Kundalini and wonder at the causes of their physical, mental, or emotional suffering or breakdown. Even those in the growth and help fields do not have easy access to information for counseling those who release extra Kundalini before their systems are ready and experience problems on all levels of life, as if 220 energy suddenly coursed through their 110 units; fuses blow and circuitry melts.

One reason for the lack of information is that many people, though knowledgeable, are concerned about the Kundalini power's potential for harm; they feel nothing should be done with it—no exercises and no training—because of the possibility that this awesome force will turn destructive. This attitude is much the same as

---

2. From the edition of W. Y. Evans-Wentz.

that of people who say that if you don't educate children about sex, there won't be any problems.

Another reason is that many people regard Kundalini as a new age fad. Nothing could be further from the truth. Kundalini can be considered the oldest known science. In previous ages people raised Kundalini under the guidance of teachers and in controlled circumstances, preserving what they learned as an esoteric knowledge. But we have entered a period of time in which the esoteric becomes exoteric.

People whose Kundalini was raised without their knowledge, relating symptoms of their condition to others, were generally considered crazy or physically weak; they may even have considered themselves crazy. The process may entail great confusion and fright beyond the exhilaration and sense of being uplifted.

It is evident from their writings that Christian mystics had experiences of released Kundalini, which they referred to as sufferings. They understood the process as one which would bring union with God.

Gopi Krishna has been a modern exponent of this evolutionary energy. His own Kundalini release came from meditation practices he undertook without prior formal training.[3] He spent years working with and understanding what was happening to him. His experiences and writings have been very beneficial to others who have not had previous training.

Symptoms of Early Release

Since we are all individuals—with our own history, physical conditions, personal and spiritual development—Kundalini release acts differently with each of us. These are some of the symptoms which may indicate an excessive release of Kundalini, meaning before the system is ready:

Unexplained illness;
Erratic behavior;
A feeling of "losing it" and difficulty coping with everyday life;
Chills or hot flashes;
Evidence of multiple personalities;
Excessive mood swings: depression or ecstasy;

---

3. See *Kundalini*, by Gopi Krishna.

Times of extreme dullness or brilliance;

Loss or distortion of memory;

Disorientation with oneself, others, work, or the world in general;

Extremes in appearance (a person may fluctuate between looking years younger one moment and twenty years older a short time later);

Visual effects: seeing lights or colors, geometric shapes, scenes from past lives, or future events.

Purpose

Kundalini has its own sense of direction. Its natural flow is up the spine and out the top of the head; along that path it brings new awareness, new abilities, and transcendental states. Much as a plant reaches toward light, the Kundalini pushes us to reach for enlightenment; it removes any energy blocks in its way, thus causing symptoms such as those listed above. It will do its own thing. We can help or hinder the process.

A fully developed person will have exceptional paranormal gifts, great spiritual awareness and truly be considered genius or God-like. Each of us must deal with the Kundalini sooner or later; the more knowledgeable and ready we are, the more wonderful the experience will be.

Chapter 2

Involuntary Release of Kundalini Energy

Process of Release

The Kundalini energy lies coiled at the base of the spine. Its release may be likened to waves, flames, pulsations or an uncoiling. The uncoiled portion seeks an outlet, normally through the spine up to the top of the head and out what is sometimes called the crown chakra. Chakra, a Sanskrit word meaning "wheel," refers to the various energy vortices on our etheric body.

Sometimes the energy coils upward around the spine, again ending at the crown chakra. In the natural evolutionary process, a number of layers or waves are individually released during a lifetime, depending on a person's growth and readiness. The movement of the wave is so imperceptible most people are not aware of the activity, though they may be aware of some heat (energy movement) in the tailbone area prior to the release. More sensitive people will feel the energy progress up the spine. They may feel pressure or pain as the energy encounters a blocked area; pain may also appear when the energy patterns are not normal.

There are many layers of Kundalini waiting to be released. The action is similar to peeling off the outer edges of an onion. A person can release a few or many layers during a lifetime. People knowledgeable about the Kundalini force may choose to release more, thus speeding their evolution; in extreme cases, liquid fire or extreme heat may be released.

The Kundalini, sometimes called *shakti* (divine spark of life

7

force), begins its ascent from the base of the tailbone, where it is stored. As it rises up the spinal column and goes out the top of the head, it blends with the spiritual energy available in the universe. An energy combination then showers down over the body and travels throughout the system, aiding in refining and cleansing the cells. If the Kundalini is blocked in its upward flow by improper energy patterns or negativity, or by an improperly prepared or cleansed body, it may drop after several days and then begin a slow, painful ascent up the body again, cleaning and refining as it goes. This process can create much havoc and may cause physical, emotional or mental distress.

A person who releases a number of layers of energy at once may be in a beautiful state for days or even weeks. Such a person may have extra physical strength, beautiful new understandings, feelings of bliss or transcendental awareness, or a feeling of really having made it and achieving enlightenment. He or she may even have a little spiritual pride. For most people, however, this state disappears and the Kundalini begins its cleansing process; then the person wonders why things are now so difficult and where the wonderful "stuff" went. The latter is the usual pattern of Kundalini release; it is not a matter of the person "messing up" their growth.

When energy blocks are severe enough, blissful states do not occur; the energy goes immediately into the cleansing. Energy blocks are caused by locked-in attitudes or feelings or old emotional or mental scars. Poor posture and injuries can also create energy blocks.

People who have prepared well by taking care of their bodies and raising spiritual awareness will accomplish Kundalini cleansing more quickly and easily; they realize benefits almost immediately and the Kundalini rising is a beautiful experience. But if the system is not ready for this powerful force, years may be required to complete the process.

Once released, there is NO TURNING BACK! It is impossible to reverse the process, though it can sometimes be slowed. If a person decides the growth is no longer desirable and tries to hold back this energy, congestion and illness may result, which may, in extreme cases, lead to death. One must learn to work with it, or in some cases just survive it, while the heavy cleansing takes place. The change is usually not a magical, total overnight operation; the energy may take as long as twenty or twenty-five years to complete cleansing

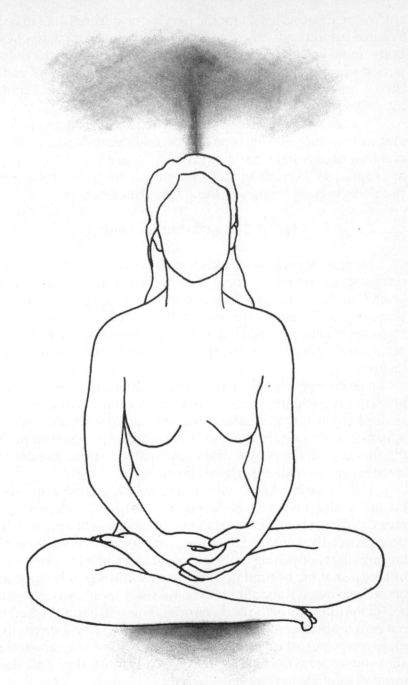

This is an example of an incorrect flow.
There is too much energy going below the person. It should all flow upwards.

and refinement sufficient for the psychic or spiritual gifts to unfold. When a person knows how to work with the energy, has a healthy body, mind and spirit and is ready, change occurs in a much shorter period of time. People in the midst of an active natural Kundalini flow, already using it, take less time to make the new Kundalini available for use.

In each incarnation it is necessary to learn over again to control and use the energy. This is one of the main purposes of childhood; children need behavior and attitude guidance to use their energies appropriately. Permitting their energies to run uncontrolled causes problems in daily living and impedes further growth.

Types of Involuntary Release

Involuntary ways in which Kundalini may be released include drug use, overwork, a severe blow or injury to the tailbone area; grief, trauma, or excessive fear; excesses in meditation, growth practices, or sex. Excessive sexual foreplay without orgasm may also cause spontaneous Kundalini release. By involuntary I do not necessarily mean unwanted; I only refer to the release of the Kundalini on its own.

The energy not only has an evolutionary purpose, it literally gives us extra energy. The body may draw from it (without our conscious knowledge) to handle extreme situations. Often, when such situations conclude, the flow continues and the person does not handle things well; the person deals now with excessive Kundalini release as well as with the original trauma.

The Aquarian Age is very intense. This intensity speeds our evolution and pushes us into a quantum leap of development in all areas. We have been very open to technological change, which has been especially incredible over the past couple decades. Now similar growth is happening in the personal and spiritual areas; we are, in fact, just at the beginning of major breakthroughs in these areas because so much Kundalini will be released spontaneously as a result of the intensity of the new energies. This will happen whether or not people are cleansed and ready. Those people who genetically are more receptive to the Kundalini and already have a fair amount useable and active will not have that much trouble; they will also be more susceptible to release.

Astrological energies play an important part in a person's

openness to extra release. A heavily aspected Uranus seems to be the cause of excessive release in some people. Saturn in the fourth house of the astrological chart may also trigger deep subconscious energies that release Kundalini. Moon in Scorpio also tends to awaken the deep subconscious energies.[1]

Some pregnant women experience extra Kundalini release from the pressure of the fetus on the Kundalini area between the anus and the genitals. Or they experience more psychic ability and awareness. Others experience postpartum depression, possibly caused by improper Kundalini flow released during the pregnancy.

People who have overworked for years may have nervous, physical, emotional, or mental breakdowns and require several months' or years' hiatus to recover; many times this, too, is attributable to excessive Kundalini pulled out by the system to handle the overload. These people later relate that their "enforced rests" were very important to them; they had time to think and change their lives. Kundalini does force us to think and change our very way of being.

Tailbone injuries may place permanent pressure upon the Kundalini reservoir, forcing a person to continually work with the energies and the changes they bring. The positive side is that the person has the extra Kundalini to force the evolutionary growth within. Grief, trauma, fear, hurtful memories all aid in "blowing open" the subconscious, which in turn releases the energies. The emotional states then usually increase out of proportion to reality and people are prone to obsession. If the extra Kundalini is not removed from the subconscious (belly area) and balanced with the rest of the body, it continues and compounds the obsessiveness. Methods which alleviate the problem through moving and balancing the energies include meditation, five to ten minutes of free form dancing (more later), or forcing oneself to think higher thoughts. Kundalini will look for the most open area or chakra to "escape" through if the body is not ready to receive its energies, blowing open a particular area or chakra and tending to pull all energies toward that spot, as if to a black hole. Only a redirection of energy releases the obsession.

Release through "recreational drugs" can be especially harmful, blowing open chakras or causing the "burnout" experienced by

1. Llewellyn's Personal Services Department offers a full range of astrological readings, described in the *New Times* magazine. See "Stay in Touch" page in the back of this book.

some drug users. The very reason some people use drugs—for paranormal experiences—may bring about a lack of paranormal ability in everyday life. A positive aspect of drug use is that users may have been opened to higher dimensions and shown mystical possibilities in life. Drug use, however, does not enable a person to achieve this state on his or her own; thus the energies are not under control, not always very useful, and sometimes exceedingly dangerous. People may have experiences but not grow in the use of their evolutionary energy.

When the excessiveness inclines toward meditation, the release of Kundalini generally goes more smoothly, as these people are already working on themselves and are open to change. Visions, mystical experiences, and excessive attention placed upon the pineal gland may also touch this reservoir of evolutionary energy and start new waves moving through the system.

Spiritual initiations from high spiritual levels are given to people who have achieved high spiritual levels in their growth. These initiations usually release at least one more layer of Kundalini. (This has nothing to do with the initiations of earthly organizations, which have their own release of Kundalini). Initiations from high spiritual levels quite often occur when a person is asleep, when there is no awareness of the event. The person only recognizes a change in perceptions and attitudes. Consciously aware of the initiation, however, a person will feel energy one could liken to a lightning bolt coming into the top of the head, which may go only as far as the heart area or all the way to the Kundalini reservoir to release some of its power. The advantage to this type of release is that there is generally more understanding of what is happening within the system. The initiation always brings greater awareness and the person does not feel as alone or crazy when the Kundalini starts doing weird things. But if the person is not physically, emotionally or mentally ready to handle the power, depression, disorientation, illness, the other problems may ensue.

Earth initiations may also trigger kundalini release. When persons have opened to higher levels (or deeper levels) of earth energy a connection (initiation) happens. This opens the person to even greater earth awareness. It comes up through the feet in a very powerful manner and goes up through the entire body and out the top of the head. If it is intense enough and the person is predisposed, the kundalini may be awakened by its power.

It is very important that people develop in all areas of life. More and more people in the counseling, religious, and medical fields are becoming acquainted with Kundalini, can recognize its symptoms, and are able to help with its process. It is an area in which all "help" and health professionals should have a working knowledge.

Symptoms of Release

Kundalini raising that occurs prior to sufficient cleansing and spiritual awareness is considered premature, producing many different symptoms. In addition to short periods of heightened awareness and states of bliss or enlightenment, there may be times of extreme dullness or depression, erratic behavior, unexplainable illness, loss of or poor memory, feelings of disorientation with oneself, friends, work or the world in general. If the liver is affected, the skin may take on a yellowish color, an almost dirty look, due to the release of negativity; or some areas of the body may take on a reddish or bluish cast. There may be other shadings relating to energy concentrations of different vibrational rates. (Each vibrational rate has its own color.) A person may look old, tired, or ill but a few hours later look years younger and full of vitality, or the reverse. Another sign of premature Kundalini raising is a blackish look to the nails of the big toes due to excessively activated reflexes in the big toes that relate to the pineal gland.

At times there may be a fluttering feeling as the muscles relax and release more energy into the nerve endings. There may be an internal fullness or pressure, a wanting to "vomit" out anything in order to release the extra energy. There may be nosebleeds. Kundalini in its stronger states can tear human tissue. There may be involuntary movements or shaking of the body; illness may ensue from Kundalini cleansings, many times remedied simply by changing the energy patterns. A warning, however: see a doctor when changing the patterns does not help; when a problem appears to be medical, do not hesitate to seek medical assistance. Symptoms are different in each individual because each person has blocks, or energy concentrations, in different areas. It is very difficult to know just how a particular person will react. One may compare the Kundalini, when a large number of waves are released all at once, to a garden hose turned on full force: if the spine is clear and straight, the force flows through to the top of the head unhampered; if blocked, twisted, or bent in some way, the free flow is stopped or hampered and the energy goes into the nearest area. A very sway-backed person, for example, will dump this energy into the belly and solar plexus area, causing intense emotions (see illustration 1 on page 15). A force that continues over a period of time may result in physical damage, stomach upsets, or even ulcers. Energy locked in the chest may make one may think of heart trouble (see illustration 2). Blockage in the brain causes loss of memory and/or mental aberrations (see illustration 3; for correct flow, see illustration 4).

Because of the varied symptoms and lack of information about Kundalini, the blame for improper and excessive release is generally misplaced. People may feel hypochondriacal with all their different aches and pains. At times they may feel ill but not actually be ill. They may feel they do not have long to live, but at the same time feel perfectly all right. Confusion is prevalent when unprepared people experience excessive Kundalini release. One woman, under a doctor's care, found she had symptoms of cancer, diabetes and heart trouble, as well as other problems, in a two year period; the symptoms later disappeared by themselves as the cleansing continued. Today she is a gifted trance reader. Another woman was ill for twenty-one years, during which time she was under the care of doctors, who finally told her they could not find her trouble and there was nothing more they knew to do for her. But when the Kundalini finished its work, she found that spiritual healing energies could flow through her hands. Misunderstandings can slow down the cleansing process and add years of concern and troubles. Cold chills or hot flashes similar to those experienced during menopause may come and go, as may psychic gifts. Change of moods, attitudes and dietary, color and style preferences are common. Some people will experience schizophrenic symptoms as the Kundalini releases energy from strong but unintegrated past-life personalities; it may be that there was little relationship between the soul and the personality and the personality remained separate, to be integrated during another life. Kundalini will seek to cleanse all locked-in memories, whether physical, emotional or mental, whether of traumatic or ecstatic events. Spontaneously or through meditations, people can relive experiences from childhood or past lives. Power trips, unexplained anger, base or perverted sexual fantasies or feelings—these are all part of personal demons, hidden away only to be brought to light by the cleansing of the Kundalini. It helps not to be afraid to

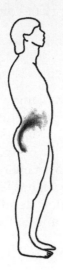

1. Emotional problems

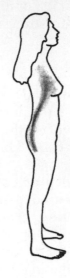

2. Heart or chest problems.

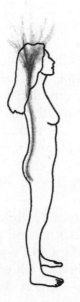

3. Mental problems.

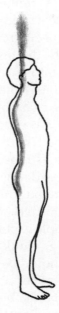

4. Correct flow.

face the memories locked within. When all blocks are released, the Kundalini flows through unhampered, refining the cells and thus allowing the prana or divine and universal energy to come into the system in pure, strong form.

Depression

Everyone who goes through Kundalini cleansing will become familiar with depression, because the energies literally lie depressed, down into the body, for our edification. Depression means something is being "dug up" for you to look at. Psychotic or chemical depression aside, plain depression concerns an energy process common to all people at some point in their lives. It has bad press in America. We need to see its positive benefits: a new depth of understanding, caring, compassion; profoundness and great creative abilities.

Enjoy your depressions! Look at this process as basically creative; *go into* the energies, exaggerate them and then listen to them. Let your mind ramble. You may remember parts of your childhood, of past lives, of recent or future events. Depression may open you to a new way of perceiving things or to new philosophical approaches. You may sense a need to change your hairstyle. You may use a new recipe, begin a new creative project; you never quite know what will come out of the depths of your subconscious. Consider depression an adventure into the deeper side of life. The subconscious does not actually like to be called the subconscious at all; it is really our *first* consciousness, a combination of physical and emotional consciousness. It is the first consciousness a baby develops, the first we as humans developed. Part of the Kundalini process is to make this first consciousness as much a part of life as mental and spiritual consciousness; in so doing its energy and information are no longer hidden or "sub" to our other levels of awareness; it becomes very useable and supportive.

Most people experience suicidal thoughts or death wishes during a cleansing. Thinking about ending life is a natural part of the process and should be recognized as such. Many old ways are dying, making way for new life. To face one's death wish with understanding can be the beginning of a new life—same body, but new spirit, and a new outlook. The process represents a release of old ways and a discovery of new ones.

Exercise of Living or Dying

As you explore your feelings about living or dying, you need to be aware whether it is you or your body that wants to call it quits. Sometimes the body is depleted or exhausted and is tired of being a vehicle; if this is the case, good nutrition, rest and better care will give you and your body a new lease on life. But if you find you have really lost the interest and motivation to live, the following may give you some new direction.

1/ In as relaxed a state as possible, meditate on all the things you have accomplished in this life; make a list and appreciate them. Then make a list of things to be accomplished. Meditate on this list also. What needs to be done to accomplish the new things?

2/ Be aware of the old patterns of your life, the old personality. What changes need to be made for a new self to emerge? What would the new personality be like in the new life? Get the feeling of the old leaving and the new coming in. The more the body feels the newness, the more quickly and easily it will make the transition. Believe that the newness is already happening.

3/ Write a news article about yourself as it might appear in the paper several years from now. It should list your accomplishments and any other things you would like to include. Meditate on different possibilities.

4/ Re-examine the death wish. Is there anything there that might give you more insight into the future?

5/ Feel again that the old way of living is leaving or dying. Let there be a rebirth into a new way of living and relating to life.

Sex and Kundalini

Sexual energy is a lower octave of the divine energy. People who accentuate their spiritual growth may be chagrined to realize that their sex drive is accentuated as well. Some people feel God is "testing" the genuineness of their desire to grow spiritually. This process is normal; when the energy of one octave is opened, the other octaves open through a resonating effect. But to keep from chasing prospective partners down the street, it would be wise to transmute some of the sexual energy into a higher form through meditation, or diffuse throughout the body and then, with mental direction, transmute it into healing, inner strength, creativity, joy, bliss, devotion, or enlightenment. Some people advocate celibacy during Kundalini raising or cleansing as a way of forcing the sexual energy to higher levels; but I think it should be each person's choice, and that choice may change quickly sometimes. The energies are intense enough during the Aquarian age that normal sex and growth can occur at the same time. If you find difficulty with whatever choice you have made, you may need to find alternatives.

During strong spiritual growth or Kundalini cleansing, past life memories may be close to the surface, resulting in attraction to people to whom you felt sexually close in a previous life. Some people feel that a sexual relationship in a previous life must be continued in this life. Not necessarily so! Be discreet and responsible with your energies; you could wear yourself out or end up in difficult relationships. If this happens to you or your spouse, don't panic! Be aware of the new influences and wait awhile before making major changes to see how the energies settle.

Affairs that begin during accelerated growth often don't last. They may be very intense, but as the song goes, "it is too hot not to cool down."[2] On the positive side, balancing the polarities of these relationships (sexual or not) can speed growth. Marriages do not have to end because one person is growing and the other does not appear to be; perhaps the other's growth is slower or in a different direction. A good marriage or relationship allows each person the freedom to develop and learn—to be on his or her own path. Always practice respect and tenderness for one another. Understanding is nice, too, but some days we don't even understand ourselves.

The strain of Kundalini experience will often speed the dissolution of a marriage or relationship that is not healthy or meant to be. In this case, the couple should work through a pre-divorce process, much as we have courtship before marriage; there needs to be loving preparation for divorce. Better to end a relationship on a positive note; you will probably meet the person again in another life!

Kundalini can affect the sexual area in a variety of ways. There may be short or prolonged periods of apathy or seeming lack of ability. There may even be frigidity, impotence, or complete lack of enjoyment. With the sexual area has been cleansed, however, the sexual energy may be transmuted and used for further cleansing and healing of the system. Sexual energy can be used for many different purposes beyond the act of sexual union: creativity, greater mental

2. From the song "Just One of Those Things" by Cole Porter.

abilities, enlightenment, inner strength and joy of life. No longer a prisoner of sexual urges or blocks, one rediscovers sex as one of life's means of expression. During Kundalini cleansing you need to accept yourself as a sexual being and recognize that the sexual energy is important to your spiritual development.

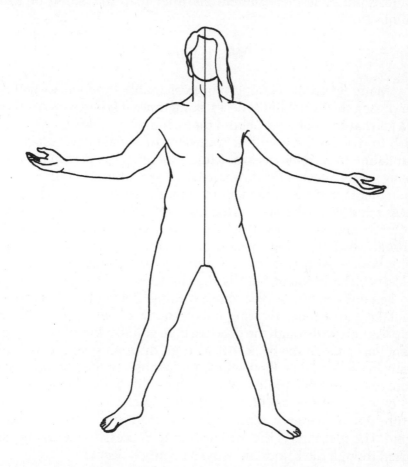

Right—Masculine Side   Left—Feminine Side

Homosexuality and lesbianism may appear as Kundalini energy brings about an androgynous state. The Kundalini forces people to deal with both masculine and feminine polarities (see illustration above). The feminine relates to the left side of the body, emotions and intuition, while the masculine relates to the right side of the body, logic and mental pursuits. Joining polarities through androgyny (developing both sides) allows high creative and spiritual forces to flow through the body; a person thus affected may experience homosexual or lesbian states for short periods of time—thoughts, feelings, and tendencies but no actions. Or this state may last for months, years, or a lifetime. There are, of course, reasons for homosexual or lesbian tendencies other than the action of Kundalini.

Weird City

Many weird or seemingly unexplainable experiences will occur during the Kundalini process. Sometimes it is best to write them in a journal and not worry about them. If they trouble you, you may wish to discuss them with a counselor or someone familiar with Kundalini. In extreme cases of Kundalini release, a person may fear losing sanity; most of the time such fear is greatly out of proportion. Then there are times when a person really doesn't care if the mind goes or not! When the stress is too high, relief from work or your everyday routine is a must. It is best to get your mind off the stress through reading, being in nature, watching television—whatever helps you. A sympathetic counselor can help you clean your inner "closets"; the problem here is that as soon as you get one thing worked out you find several more waiting. Remember, this process can take a long time. Treating it as a course in basic humanity can help. As you go through the process, give yourself lots of encouragement and pats on the back. All who go through strong Kundalini cleansing will change their whole philosophy of life and how they want to live out that philosophy. It is possible to experience a number of waves of Kundalini, to go through a cleansing and then at a future date experience more release and go through the process again. The first time is the most difficult. Successive cleansings are easier, though the Kundalini waves go much deeper.

Living in the World during Cleansing

Life is much more difficult for those caught in the nine-to-five workday world because finding time to work with the Kundalini process is a challenge. But unless you regularly find time, you may find you contract the "Kundalini flu," wherein energies get so backed up in your system as to cause aches, pains, or flu-like symptoms. You are genuinely sick enough to stay home from work. Lying in bed allows the Kundalini free rein to work through your system. You feel better or are well when it is done.

But there are many things you can do besides lie in bed to facilitate correct, unhampered flow of Kundalini (whether only one or two waves have been released or a larger amount). One purpose of Kundalini is to cleanse and refine the body cells so that higher mental and spiritual energies can operate in the system. Anything which aids in this process is of benefit. Learning to be aware of where the energy is, where it wants to go, and helping its movement all shorten cleansing time and lessen pain and confusion. It may only be a matter of giving in to thoughts and feelings and letting them work through; or it may involve moving the energy, through thought control or visualization, from an excessive area back to the spine and up and out the top of the head (see Mixing and Showering Technique, page 178). Releasing pressure from an affected area promotes healing. If you are working outside the home and don't have control of your time, you can take lunch hours and breaks just to tune into your system, center energies and relax; a few minutes here and there in the day can be very helpful. Also take time for reflection and energy exercises before or after work. Write down your thoughts, feelings, and experiences; try to take at least an hour a day.

Some marriages are irreparably strained during one partner's Kundalini cleansing. Spouses who stay the storm of erratic moods and powerful energies are to be commended. Sometimes the Kundalini release in one triggers a partner's release; this indicates that the couple has to grow and open to new possibilities of life (not each in the same way, but as individuals). It should be mentioned that not all marriages that end during a Kundalini cleansing do so because of a spouse's Kundalini process.

Associates, co-workers and friends may not understand what is happening to you. Spare them long definitions and treatises. You will still seem rather obsessed and maybe a little crazy to them anyway. Explain you are going through energy work and let it be. Those who are knowledgeable about the process may know the right questions to ask and then share something from their own experience. I excused the heaviest symptoms of my own release on menopause and low-blood sugar. I was menopausal age, after all, and did have some low-blood sugar problems; the symptoms were similar and such an explanation stemmed a lot of useless explanation. In any event, returning to as simple and plain a life as possible is practically a necessity. Eliminating unnecessary outside activities may not only be helpful but mandatory. Taking part in activities which ask only a little attention of you may relax you and allow the body processes to continue more or less on their own. There are times to be aware of the cleansing and times to ignore it.

Getting caught up too intensely in the process slows progress. Remain objective and avoid morbidity. Remember that Kundalini cleansing is a natural process. During excessive release, it may indeed be much more noticeable and difficult to live with. Be prepared for anything to happen during the cleansings: radical changes in personality, spirituality, or in any level of being. Still, you need to function in your world, so retain a modicum of control. Time in Nature is very beneficial. Creative pursuits and music are important parts of the unfolding. Good health practices are a must; your system is going through enough strain. Chemicals are difficult for the body to digest, so try to avoid preservatives, artificial colorings and flavorings. It may help to eat smaller, more frequent meals, six to eight per day in severe cases. This eases digestion and slows the whole process. Unnecessary drugs only increase the load the system has to handle. Needless worry and concern also add to the load, while understanding and acceptance of the process are most helpful.

You may crave foods that promote releasing the emotional content of blocked energy. As much as possible, however, maintain a balanced diet. Occasional "junk" food when energy is too high can be helpful in slowing the process. Each person must judge what is best. (My cure for constipation caused by the Kundalini release was to eat brownies and dill pickles together.) It is important to get in touch with what works. Get plenty of rest—more than usual; it need not be sleep (many people find it very difficult to sleep during cleansings), but rest for the entire system is essential.

Physical exercise is a must, whether you feel up to it or not. In extreme cases, where there does not seem to be enough energy for even the mildest exercise, try simple stretching exercises, in bed or on the floor. Peaceful, deep breathing is very helpful. Dancing, especially free-form, walking, bicycling and swimming all help keep the energy flowing and also break down the blocks. Exercises such as yoga, tai chi and judo, aid energy flow and release blocks in the system. During excessive release, however, moderate these exercises, if you do them at all, as they have a tendency to produce even greater Kundalini release. Osteopathic and/or chiropractic treatments can keep the spine aligned and make the flow easier. Massage is an excellent way to release blocked energy and move energies which are already unblocked but not yet fully released from the body. During massage, let the mind ramble and feelings come to the awareness. Deep muscle work may be helpful for some people, releasing the more intense blocks, causing release not only on the physical level but on the emotional, mental and (sometimes) spiritual levels. Here, however, one may find that so much energy is freed in such a short period of time that concerns mount and the whole situation becomes even more difficult to handle. A system blocks energy because of the person's fear of handling it. Sudden release sometimes brings more energy than is helpful, old structures leaving so fast that a person may have trouble knowing how or where to relate in the new state, even to the point of trying to put the block back. When too much Kundalini is released in the process, professional counseling may be in order.

Some people experience itching at some point in Kundalini release, either in localized areas of the skin or over the entire body. Massaging lotions into the skin may help. During an extreme amount of cleansing, daily or more frequent baths or showers are very beneficial.

A very real concern in Kundalini cleansing is lack of understanding of what is taking place. Through misunderstanding or lack of courage, one may try to block feelings rather than face them and let them be cleansed. Granted this may occur unconsciously, but any attempts to block or close the energy flows or cleansing may cause the energy to reverse and lock into certain areas with severe and sometimes disastrous results. In extreme cases, people are bedridden for years. If the Kundalini goes down instead of up there may be great trouble with the legs, including temporary paralysis. A downward flow may also result in tremendous negativity. A common symptom of Kundalini cleansing is disorientation—the feeling that one is not connected and that nothing will give a feeling of stability or security. Since cleansing removes all the old blocks and patterns and makes room for a new energy flow, it is no wonder that there is disorientation; it is similar to gutting and totally rebuilding a house. Sometimes it's painful!

You may be forced to understand events in a different light or forgive yourself and others in order to complete the release. Shallow understanding and a lack of love cause more rigid blocks than other human deficiencies such as fear, ego and greed. Sometimes exaggerating the sensation or emotion may promote release, giving a person a feeling of control and at the same time bringing more awareness to the situation.

The Kundalini cleansing is essentially a journey of the self, but it is not for the self alone. Your energies will help other people grow and be more evolved. You need to have a support system available, not to take over your part in the process, but simply to help.

- Faith is one of the most important ingredients for a successful Kundalini cleansing process
- Faith that it is a process, which with some attention and guidance will do very well
- Faith that it has its own purpose, which is your elevation
- Faith in yourself that you will bounce back from whatever you have to go through
- Faith in a supreme or divine being who does know and care about what you are going through.

Prayer and devotional energies can alleviate much of the burden. One day you will look back and say that every bit of it was worth it.

Exercises for Handling Involuntary Release

The following exercises can be used by anyone, whether extra Kundalini is flowing or not. They are primarily for cleansing and refining. Some help develop control of energies. When a particular exercise releases too much energy, do not repeat it until the new energy is integrated into the system.

Have a friend lead the exercises, as it is much easier to "get into" an exercise when you don't have to read during the procedure. If no one is available to help, you can put the instructions on tape.

When time or attention is limited, the following four exercises can provide much assistance over a short period.

Deep, Peaceful Breathing
Relax your body as much as possible while keeping your back

straight. Lying down is the best position. Breathe deeply and slowly the way the system wants. If abdominal breathing is easiest, do that; if chest breathing, do that. Do whatever is most peaceful so that the concentration is not on the mechanics. (This exercise tends to correct many breathing problems naturally.)

Let the breaths go deep into the body, deep into each cell. If the breathing pattern begins to change, let it. Let the body choose what it wants. See the energy of the breath going into each cell. This exercise is excellent whether done for a few minutes or half an hour. It is also excellent before meditations, during the day as a refresher, or as a relaxer before sleeping.

Mental Control

Learning to control the flow and direction of body energy will greatly reduce concentrations. Here are three ways to do it:

1/ Be aware of any area in the system which seems blocked and let energy radiate from there to the entire body.

2/ Be aware of any area which seems blocked and "think" the energy back to the spine, up and out the top of the head.

3/ Be aware of any area which is tense and "think" extra energy into the tenseness to help break through and release it.

Open Meditation

Do the Deep, Peaceful Breathing for a few minutes. Concentrate your attention on any area of the body causing pain or feeling blocked. Massaging the area also helps. Let your attention wander to anything it wishes. Situations, feelings or thoughts will usually come to mind which pertain to the troubled area; simply observe them and how the body feels. Do not try to stop them. If tears come, let them. Releasing blocked thoughts and feelings can be accomplished in as little as five to fifteen minutes, or it may take as much as an hour. When new energy floods the system there is often sense of peacefulness.

Cleansing Screen

Lie down and do the Deep, Peaceful Breathing for a few minutes. Imagine lying on a screen that is larger than your physical body. Slowly visualize or imagine the screen rising up through your body, cleansing all negativity and removing blocks. When that is done, pray that the energy of the negativity and blocks be turned back into pure energy and released into the universe for the good of all. You may first wish to observe the blocks and ponder their symbolism.

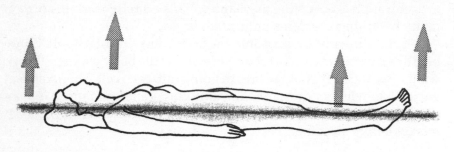

The imaginary cleansing screen goes up through the body, removing blocks.

Broccoli

(This exercise is called the broccoli because the energy looks much like stalks of broccoli.) Choose an area of your body that feels sluggish or is causing a problem. Imagine that this area is full of broccoli-colored energy and is rather solid in appearance. Then visualize the part nearest the surface of the skin as being made up of green bubbles, similar to the top of broccoli flowers; imagine or visualize the bubbles turning to a light green, then to a gold as the energy is released out through the skin. The changing of the colors resembles the ripening of the broccoli tops. A general energy release can be achieved by starting with the liver, and proceeding to the pancreas, stomach, heart, intestines or any other area you desire.

Spinal Relaxation

This is for relaxing the "super-highway" or "communications channel." Lie down, placing your arms above your head on the floor. Pull knees to chest. Feel your spine touch the floor; let it relax, let it go. Let the tension drop into the floor. Be aware where tension persists and massage each of those areas. If possible, have someone massage your back. Repeat the exercise. Spend five to ten minutes in a meditative state.

Breathing Exercises

One of the most important things to consider, in or outside Kundalini cleansing, is breathing. There are many variations of breathing exercises depending on the purpose. The following are a few of the possibilities. Be careful, as the more advanced breathing techniques may release Kundalini in unmanageable ways.

Color Breathing. Sit or lie comfortably, making sure your spine is straight. Begin to breathe into the whole body, feeling the breath enter each cell, then imagine that your body is filled with a red light (make it a red "with love" so it does not bring up old frustrations). Hold this for a few minutes, breathing it into each cell, aware of the vibrational quality in the system. Release the red light and do the same with orange, yellow, green, blue, purple and lavender (in that order). Finally, fill the body with a radiant white light and meditate on the divine source. (The meditation can be varied by focusing on God, a spiritual being, the universe, the purpose of life or a spiritual verse or idea.) After finishing the exercise, stretch your entire body.

Vibrational Breathing. Sit erect or lie comfortably, spine straight. Breathe deeply, allowing the entire chest and abdominal regions to protrude. First, fill the lower part of the chest with air, extending the abdomen slightly, then expand the middle of the chest and finally the upper part of the chest. Inhale for seven counts; hold for seven counts, exhale to the count of seven, and hold the breath out for seven counts. Repeat. You may synchronize your counting with your pulse beat; speed doesn't matter as much as evenness and continuity.

If your chest barely moves during inhalation or exhalation, try consciously pushing it out while inhaling and pulling it in while exhaling. Many people's rib cages are so locked in by their muscle system that it is difficult for them to take a good breath. As the rhythm gets going and the counting becomes automatic, become aware of the pulse of the universe—its in and out movement—and its vibrational hum. You may follow this exercise with open meditation.

Freeing Breathing. Take deep, peaceful breaths. Concentrate on your breath leaving your toes, then your fingers, then the top of your head. Visualize or imagine your breath taking the tensions of life with it as it leaves these areas.

This is an excellent exercise for equalizing the energy in the body and thereby relaxing the system. It brings a refreshed feeling, especially when followed by at least five to ten minutes of rest.

Complete Breathing. This is called complete breathing because when done correctly the breathing cycle fills the entire system. At first, practice it lying down. Bend your knees so that your feet are flat on the floor; place your hands—fingertips barely touching—on the belly below your navel. On the inhalation, separate your fingers slightly. When you gain some skill, try this breathing sitting up, then in a standing position. It should eventually become the normal way to breathe. There are six steps:

1/ Fill the lower part of your lungs, allowing your diaphragm to extend and the abdominal wall to expand.

2/ Fill the middle of the lung area, allowing your rib cage to extend.

3/ Fill the top of the lungs, allowing your upper chest to extend and the abdominal wall to recede. Pulling the abdominal wall back in allows the top of the lungs to fill more completely. (Note: perform the above three steps in one continuous movement using six pulse beats.)

4/ Hold your breath for a few seconds, allowing your chest and belly to relax more fully.

5/ Exhale slowly and evenly, pulling and lifting your abdomen, allowing your chest to contract; do this using six pulse beats.

6/ Allow your chest and abdominal areas to relax and be still for a few seconds before beginning the process over again. Be sure your back is also relaxed.

Make sure when standing or sitting that your chest is very erect; slouching will not allow the lungs to fill properly. This is not easy at first; it will take practice and patience. Two or three complete breaths are enough in the beginning. Gradually increase the number until ten FULL complete breaths can be done with no strain.

Cleansing Breathing. First, do three complete breaths (see above exercise), holding the breath for several seconds on the third complete breath. Second, holding your cheeks firmly, pucker your lips and force breath out in short blasts, holding briefly in between each blast. Continue until all air is expelled. The force of each "blast" helps cleanse the system and revitalize it. Repeat, taking only one complete breath for each exhalation.

Flute Breathing. Do the above exercise but on the exhalation hold your lips as if playing a flute or blowing over a bottle top. Keep the exhalation in one continuous stream until all air is expelled. This releases excess energy.

Chapter 3

Daily Routine

A daily routine helps a person stay centered and prevents new blocking of the Kundalini as it races through the body. It also gives you the feeling of doing something, of being in some kind of control. Daily routines also help stabilize any "weirdness."

It is best if you design your own daily routine to fit your personal needs. Below are some suggestions; modify them or make any changes you deem necessary.

You may think of disciplining yourself to follow your daily routine. However, discipline is imposing form and structure upon yourself. This is in direct opposition to the Kundalini, which opts for more flowing and results in motivation: doing things because you "want to" rather than the "have to" of discipline. A person's daily routine will then have much greater benefit because energy is flowing rather than being forced. If you have trouble in getting motivated, you might try imagining yourself doing the exercises or other parts of the routine. This puts the energy into the body, and as it seeks expression motivation will automatically be there.

Exercise

Some type of physical activity is imperative when Kundalini has released. It is necessary to keep energy moving, thus preventing new blocks and concentrations of energies which cause bleeding, pain, or other physical problems. People should decide individually what physical exercise is most helpful. I have found that slow, graceful stretching combined with deep, peaceful breathing is very beneficial. I have also found free form dancing to be exceptionally helpful.

Free Form Dancing

In free form dancing the body helps with the dance through expression of feelings, thoughts, or body sensations. Everyone's style is different because what each person works with is different. If you feel uncomfortable dancing, you may wish to lock your bedroom door or wait until no one else is home. Many people (especially men) feel quite inhibited with free form movement; they may prefer Tai Chi, an ancient Chinese form of energy movement, incredibly effective in releasing and moving energy. Some people may find that dancing releases too much too fast and need to go a little slower with it.

Free form dancing generally includes a lot of arm movement, bringing energy releases and great changes in the body. Tightening and hunching the shoulders, you control energy in your body and hold back expression, which arm movement automatically releases.

At first most people feel comfortable moving only the upper part of the body; but be sure to include the bottom half of your body as well. Many people feel bound up or restricted by their bodies and wish to be free of them. They forget they added the restrictions in the first place, whether through blocking expression or creating body tension through fear, excessive worry or overwork. We can learn to feel great freedom through the body.

Vary your music selections; different types work differently. If no music is available, you may wish to "sound" the feelings inside you. In sounding, make whatever noise wishes to come out. An alternative is to "sound" or feel an imaginary rhythm.

Other aids in getting started include dancing while sitting down, stretching as a dance form, or lying down and daydreaming the dance prior to dancing.

Variations

1/ Guide your awareness to the superficial facia (the area just under the skin all over the body). Continued awareness will release the energy in the facial system, influencing the dance. This is extra-beneficial for circulation.

2/ Imagine yourself in a different time period, wearing clothing suitable to that period. You may wish to use music corresponding to the mood you are creating. Scenes or memories may come spontaneously as you dance. You may even release blocks from that time; blocks do sometimes carry over into the present life.

3/ Dancing with a partner or partners can mutually enhance energy release.

Energy Exercises

Some form of structured energy movement each day or every other day is very helpful in training yourself to be aware of energy and to control its movement. Below are two suggestions. If you release too much energy with these exercises, slow down or eliminate them for awhile until your body catches up with the energy changes.

1/ The basic Kundalini and Chakra exercise on page 55. This can be done very quickly as an energy exercise, or more slowly if you wish to spend more time developing Chakras.

2/ Basic *Sushumna* (main Nadi located in the spine, see page 166). Put your awareness on *Sushumna*, in the middle of your spine. Feel it open and free. Breathe peacefully and deeply into *Sushumna*, and also around it, visualizing the entire area bathed in light (see Color Plate 4).

Variations

a/ Visualize a silver light (spiritual) and at other times a golden light (high mental); this develops both energies and keep them in balance.

b/ Use rainbow colored lights, one at a time, as a means of learning to change the frequencies of energy even further. This gives the self more flexibility and the ability to "shift gears" as the day demands. One problem many people have in this fast paced, changing world is not being flexible enough to roll with what happens and make necessary changes. This variation helps keep you from becoming crabby or stressed with the day's tension.

c/ While dancing, concentrate on any blocked or tight areas. You may wish to let that energy expand over the entire body, bringing lightness and a sense of freedom.

d/ Sitting or lying down, expand the energy from *Sushumna* to all of the cells in the body, bringing light to them.

e/ Throughout, include any prayers or mantras you wish.

f/ While visualizing the energy in and around *Sushumna* and throughout your body, visualize what you will do the next day (if you do the exercise in the morning, visualize the day's activities). This makes your work more balanced and effective.

g/ Visualizing the energy in and around *Sushumna* and throughout your body, lift up your chest and take deep, peaceful breaths; this aids in cleansing and refining the body. Also be aware of your chakras flowing and glowing.

h/ Think of the spine, the most important super-highway for Kundalini flow. Maintain plenty of space for the nerves to carry on their communicating work. Blood vessels in this area also use this infrastructure. The entire system works better when the spine is in "good shape."

i/ Doing any of these variations outdoors can open you to a new awareness of nature. Exercising outdoors at least once a season helps keep you in the rhythm of life.

j/ Standing outdoors, visualize gold and silver energy in and around *Sushumna* radiating outwards. Add an awareness of this energy going deeply into the Earth, and steeply into the Heavens, increasing your feeling of connection with eternity while you are very presently here.

k/ While doing (d), balance overall growth by spending some time in awareness of your physical body, then of your emotional, mental and spiritual levels.

l/ Also while doing (d), be aware of your right and left sides, including right and left brains; feel them in balance. Visualize a very open *corpus colossum* (bridge between your two brains); feel the light in *Sushumna* balancing and blending the right and left energies. This promotes creativity and leaves you centered.

m/ After visualizing *Sushumna* full of light, let that light expand to the entire body and visualize all of the Nadis as open and radiant; there are thousands of them in the body which together form an etheric nervous system that has the potential to vivify the entire body and chakras.

n/ Use (d) briefly several times during the day as a centering meditation, bringing an inner strength and flow appropriate to the day's activities.

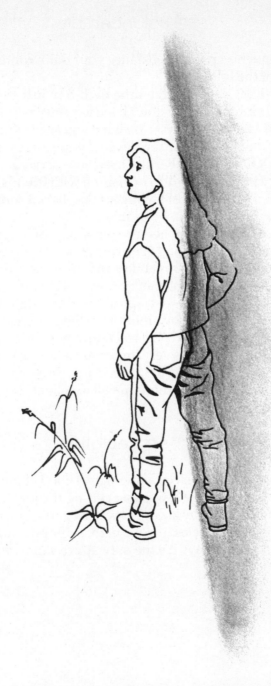

Variation J—let the energies expand to heaven and earth.

Balanced Life

As much as possible, balance your daily routine; include time on each of the following:

a/ BEING—take some time each day just to let go of everything and simply be. You don't have to justify yourself, prove yourself, or explain yourself; you are what you are. It's good to take a few moments and BE who you are (even if you're not sure who you are).

b/ DOING—whether it's exercise, carrying out the garbage, planning a big financial deal or visiting with friends, DO something. We all need the feeling of having accomplished something. DOING also trains our energy to be usable.

c/ LEARNING—whether something of importance to your life or something you don't even care about, take the time to LEARN something; expand the capability and usefulness of your brain. In a well functioning system, energy flows well through the brain.

d/ INSPIRITING—let spirit flow through you every day, whether through love, joy, union with Divine, creativity or bliss. Inspiriting is an important physical nourishment for our systems and creativity in particular is very important as an expression of the new Kundalini; journaling, writing, doodling, drawing or painting, photography, building collections are all excellent ways to express this energy.

Appreciation

Before you go to sleep at night, feel good about something that you have done, even if it was just getting through the day. You are the only one who really knows how hard you work, the stress you're under and the obstacles in your path; self-appreciation is very important and some days it's the only appreciation you get!

Chapter 4

The Seven Body
Approach to Growth

There are seven basic vibratory rates (bodies) which we use to progress from very basic energies to the very highly developed superhuman levels. These bodies interpenetrate one another, the higher bodies extending further out. There are levels beyond the seven, but we will not work with them in this book because they are useable only by the very advanced.

The densest of these bodies, and the only one readily seen, is the physical. The other bodies, vibrating at correspondingly higher rates, are the emotional, mental, intuitional, atmic (atma means great self), monadic (monad is a unit), and divine. A man or woman, however, is not these seven bodies; each is rather a pure consciousness which can reside in any one or a combination of bodies. There are very few people in this particular age whose consciousness is so developed, their bodies so vivified and attuned, that they function in all bodies at once; but this is nonetheless the ultimate goal of earthly development. A person functioning in all bodies at once—that is, all bodies in harmony with his or her consciousness—lives as perfect a life as is possible on this earth.

Most people interact with others and the world only through a few of their bodies. A person may be primarily physical/emotional or physical/mental or perhaps mental/spiritual. Aquarian Age energies push for balance and synthesis of all bodies; no matter whether or not you are interested in Kundalini, you have to work with your different bodies or levels of consciousness.

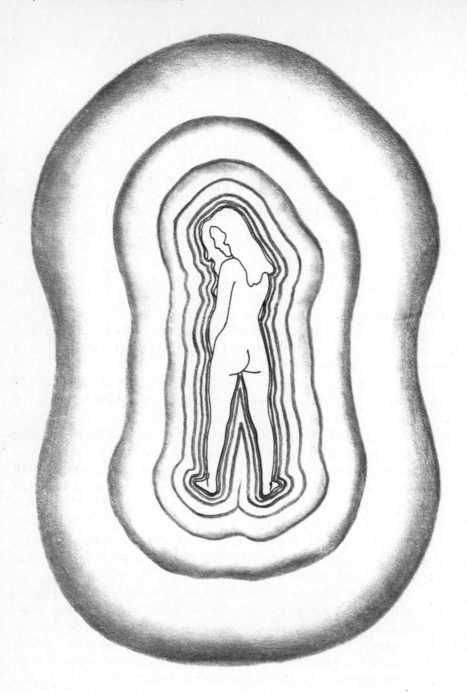

Our seven levels of consciousness (bodies) extend way beyond our physical bodies.

The Three Personality Bodies

The Physical Body

The physical body is a living machine through which our higher bodies express themselves. In blocking off your physical body, so do you block the expressions of your higher self. You can feel or think a good deal, but if you deny physical expression or action you become frustrated and subject to further problems. Problems which manifest in the physical body as aches, pains, or illness are simply the result of blocks preventing the expression of higher bodies.

The physical body is composed of cells marked by their own individuality. We should not keep these cells under a conscious control or dominating control, but a loving one. If one considers the physical body as a universe unto itself, each of us is "god" of our own universe. The physical body has two parts, the dense and the etheric; the etheric is very closely connected with our nervous system.

Cleansing the Physical

One can use Kundalini on the physical level to achieve a healthier body. The technique of directing Kundalini having been learned, energy may be sent to different areas of the body for rejuvenation, healing and strengthening. Working with it, one develops a sense of how much to send to each area and how it works best. The exercise for Kundalini Movement and Chakra Cleansing on page 55 is excellent for understanding how to guide the energy.

Letting the Kundalini flow gently into the area needing healing—changing it to the quality of liquid silk—is very soothing; the frequency of the energy changes to one more conducive to general healing. Bathe a particular area in this energy. Next, diffuse the energy throughout the entire body. Several sessions a week will increase circulation, help release blocks and generally aid in maintaining a youthful body.

Faced with a need for greater than normal physical exertion, fill your body with the power of Kundalini; breathe it throughout the entire body, let it flow through and then do the task. Practice with it to see how to handle and use it.

When physically affected by the various aches and pains stemming from raised Kundalini effect, promote release with deep, peaceful breathing followed by massage in the affected area; allow thoughts and feelings to come to your consciousness. Such an open meditation can be most helpful. If you cannot, for some reason, massage the hurt area (perhaps it is too painful), focus your attention on that area instead; concentrate your energy there and go into the discomfort. Often the aches and pains will leave in a short while and you will develop a memory or awareness of what has occurred.

The Ultimate

The physical body, cleansed and refined by the Kundalini, will appear youthful and be very energetic. It will seldom be ill (or illness will be short), have great power, and be capable of paranormal feats.

The Emotional Body

Our feelings emanate from the emotional body. We feel anger there, frustration when our needs are not met. From the emotional body we learn to give and express love and caring, thus fulfilling our needs to be in relationships. The emotional body is very demanding; seeking fulfillment, if not directly, through various hidden ways. Feeling depleted or unable to express, it may seek gratification and balance in smoking, eating certain foods, irrational behavior or any number of other ways. When we keep direct contact with our emotions we can deal with these in better ways.

Cleansing the Emotional

As the Kundalini cleanses the emotional area, one may find that emotions are out of proportion to a given situation. There may be crying spells or other emotional states without apparent reason; the Kundalini is simply hitting a block full-force. One's usual reaction is to block again; it is much better to enter an open meditation, allowing thoughts and feelings to surface, thus letting the block release. The block may be related to the feeling level either of a past life or an earlier experience from this life. It may also represent a present problem. Sometimes it even relates to things which have not yet happened but have only begun to manifest through the system.

Emotional Control

Emotions and feelings are just vibratory rates; changing the rates, we can change our emotions and feelings. As an exercise, feel your sadness as deeply as possible. Now turn the sadness to joy and try to notice a change of vibrational quality. Do the same with fear, turning it into faith and courage. Feel jealousy; turn that into understanding your own needs. Turn pride into thankfulness. Take any emotional quality that is difficult for you, think of its opposite, and work with it in this manner.

Learn to feel without getting caught in it. Keep a perspective on the situation by equalizing energies in the body. Feel energy in the back as well as the front; energy that remains primarily in the belly area creates a tendency in us to give far more attention to the feelings than they deserve. Massage the belly area and ask what is there that needs to be recognized; then move the energy into the entire body, to assimilate or eliminate it.

The Ultimate

After cleansing and refining, it is possible to have feelings without getting caught in them, to experience life without causing more karma and blocks, and to love without attachment. The emotional body will then give richness and depth to whatever you do.

The Mental Body

The mental body contains matter which can vibrate at a rate similar to that of the creative force in our cosmos. It is where we begin to think, to reason, to know, to create. Through the mental body we gather knowledge; through reason and logic, we apply that knowledge. It is also through this body that we set up rigid attitudes or structures in our system. Here prejudices are formed. The more rigid the matter in our mental body becomes, the more difficult it is to flow with life, to learn new ways of living and to acquire new ideas.

Cleansing the Mental

While the Kundalini cleanses the mental body, a person may find strong, previously unknown prejudices or become aware of life-governing attitudes which have long determined actions and reactions.

Clearing the Brain

Concentrate on breathing through your nose, up into your head. Look into your head as you would look up into the heavens and observe the stars in the sky. What colors, what energy patterns can you observe?

Truth

Do the Deep, Peaceful Breathing, concentrating on the center of your forehead; visualize the word "truth" in that area. Breathe in and feel truth enter your entire system, flooding each cell. Try to hold this in the system, while doing the Deep, Peaceful Breathing, for at least two minutes.

During Kundalini cleansing it is especially easy for untruths and misconceptions (which block growth) to enter your thoughts. If you have mental work to do but your energy will not flow, try dancing. Dancing is excellent for releasing Kundalini flow and will aid in the thinking and intuitive processes. Since mental work is often done in a way that is not conducive to good Kundalini flow—at a desk or a table, curved over your work, shoulders rounded and hunched, head lowered—try to improve your posture and take breaks in which you walk, dance or exercise.

Kundalini flow to the brain is slowed when you are caught in emotional situations and relationship problems (common, in this age). Having faith that "this too shall pass," and gaining perspective on the situation, helps keep energy flow open to the brain.

The Ultimate

You will think and create in new ways and work with higher dimensions. Manifestation and other mental powers will be considered normal.

The Four Spiritual Bodies

The Intuitional/Compassionate Body

This is the first of the four bodies of our spiritual self. It serves as a balance between the personality and other spiritual bodies. It is also a vehicle for contact with the universal mind that brings insights and understandings to our human level. It is the source of ideas resulting from abstract thinking or awaring (as opposed to the concrete logical thinking of the mental body). The intuitional/compassionate body also relates to understanding (really only another word for compassion). It is sometimes called the Buddhic body, after the compassionate Buddha.

During development of this body, intuition may wax and wane. It is difficult at times to determine the accuracy of received information, but holding the energy of the intuition in the body can help you decide. When it resonates deep inside the self, it is usually right. Be patient as you learn how to use it.

Cleansing the Intuitional/Compassionate

Kundalini flowing through this body may result in an overabundance of compassion. A person may be overcome with love for others and for the world. Negative energy may take the form of self pity. In any event, these feelings are usually out of proportion. To relieve the excess energy, allow your system to feel light and floating. Lie down; fill yourself with a light blue color and maintain a feeling of floating for approximately thirty minutes. This will help balance the energies.

This Too Shall Pass

Understand that what is happening is temporary and that there is a purpose to being cleansed and refined. Be aware of your depths of despair, disillusionment, depression, or whatever your experience is, and breathe into it. Next go into it deeply until you come to the "silver lining," or break through to peace and joy.

Suffering is the Other Side of Joy

Suffering stretches us, allowing new understanding to come through and new energy to flow in. Fill your body with a taffy color. Courageously and faithfully, let your feelings of suffering be stretched and opened until joy and peace flow in.

Spiritual Breathing
Breathe into the top part of your lungs; feel expansion. Be uplifted by this beautiful energy. This helps activate spiritual centers, reducing excess energy in the emotional and mental areas and helping clear and cleanse.

The Ultimate
We will live by intuition, awareness, and insight. We will love and feel compassion without getting caught in other people's "stuff." There will be a beautiful balance between the human and spiritual aspects of life. There will be a new understanding of God and the universe.

The Atmic Body (or Will/Spirit)

Kundalini is very at home in the will/spirit body. By its very nature, Kundalini needs to flow, and this body is one of flowing, moving, and acting. It is extremely easy to get carried away with this flow. More karma is created through the incorrect use or non-use of the will/spirit than through the other bodies; this energy has a much stronger quality and needs plenty of direction. On the positive side, a person can have great charisma and feel bliss or rapture states.

Cleansing the Will/Spirit
As cleansing progresses to the will/spirit level, you may get involved in power trips, common among which are thinking you have the answers to every problem and thinking that personal power is unlimited, whether political or financial, charm, handsomeness or beauty. In general, such a power trip indicates excessive ego and an excessive use of will.

Personality Changes
Keeping an even flow of energy on the atmic level is extremely difficult. People who have had rather weak or quiet personalities may find themselves totally changed through the Kundalini cleansing, even to the point of going through Jekyll/Hyde transitions, very charming sometimes and almost demonic at others.

Attachments

Everything is accelerated through Kundalini. Do not get too caught up in what is happening. Attachments to actions, ideas, thoughts, guilt, pride, and feelings may cause blocks and a good deal of wasted energy. Let loose of your shoulders and hips and relax your body. Are you using your will/spirit well, or are there other choices?

Not My Will, but Thine

Think of how often in the past few days you have used your will to get things done. Have the uses been wise? Be in prayer. Ask to know God's will for yourself. Do not fight God's will but join your personal will with it.

The Ultimate

The will/spirit body is the home of sex and is where our male and female (positive and negative) polarities are separated. (They are joined in the soul level body.) In the ultimate energy, these polarities are balanced and very useable. Balance will align us with evolution and divine will. Great powers, joy, and bliss will be natural parts of our being.

The Monadic Body (or Soul Level)

Monad is Greek for "unit." The monadic body expresses the unity of the polarities and allows the soul to express itself in the physical body.

Cleansing the Monadic

At times, through the action of Kundalini, one has contact with the soul and feels pure and holy. At other times one has no concept of any soul. Feelings alternate between one-with-all and complete isolation. The monadic is one of the most difficult areas to clean because it touches our essence, our whole way of being.

With poor energy flow at the monadic or soul level, you may feel you have no right to exist; this in turn may lead to feeling apologetic for everything that happens to others, as if somehow you are the cause of others' problems. The monadic is also the level of true career and services, where much of the purpose of life is determined (after taking into account the karmic forces active on all levels). It is the synthesizer of the karmic energy from past lives.

Universal Exercise

Enter a meditative state and feel your soul-self as a cell in the body of God. Continue the meditation for five to ten minutes, in tune to any messages you might receive.

This Moment of Eternity

Enter a meditative state, aware of your soul in this moment of eternity. Hold that concept and feeling for at least five minutes; it can bring a great sense of peace, connectedness, and universality.

The Ultimate

When the monadic body is developed, your sense of I AMness or soul awareness is so strong that the "I" can merge with the divine, be one with all and experience both states (the I and the Thou). You radiate inner peace and understand your purpose and existence. The essence of the soul shines through your eyes.

The Divine Body

Kundalini in the divine body enables a person to feel oneness with God and the cosmos, to be in touch with his or her own spark of God consciousness, to feel divine energy and love in life. As the monadic synthesizes our individual karmic energy, so the divine level synthesizes our individual karmic energy with the karmic energy pervading everything, whether from families, friends, communities, nations, ideas, social pressures, the forces from the geographical areas in which the individual lives, forces from planets, stars— any other force. We are all very much affected by these other forces, whether we realize it or not.

Cleansing the Divine

At the divine level a person's concept of God and the universe changes more radically that at other levels. Many go through the "dark night of the soul," doubting God, existence, purpose or anything else in life. The divine body receives both the most traumatic and most rewarding cleansing and refinement. Those with strong faith in a Divine Being have an easier time on this level; even during times of disbelief, they have some faith to sustain them.

Facing Demons

Facing demons is necessary. At times you may be totally against the spiritual side of life, whether on account of feeling separate from God or actually experiencing the demons which need to be transformed. A person in the midst of cleansing is very aware of this demonic side, which may involve deep feelings of bitter hatred, sexual perversion, sadism, or other unacceptable tendencies. Pray for strength and guidance as you confront your demons. Fill yourself with a light lavender; breathe deeply and peacefully. Let your cells be cleansed, transformed, and filled with spiritual energy. By doing so you will redeem the negative forces within, "save" yourself from the negative. It is only by facing the demons and transmuting their energy that we eradicate them; some people prefer professional counseling when dealing with this aspect of life.

Voids

Focus and meditate on any area of your body. Imagine that the area is a void, empty of all but spiritual energy; then imagine your entire system is a void, open to being filled with spiritual energies. Many people are so afraid of emptiness that they fill it with anything, thus complicating life.

Presence of God

Feel the presence of God all around. Know that God is within and without at all times. Just being aware of the Presence allows it to enter.

The Ultimate

Developing the divine body enables you to know God's will for you and be open to cosmic or Christ consciousness. We can use this cosmic energy in our everyday lives. It opens us to living in constant oneness with God.

Synthesizing the Bodies

Each body has its own function and sense of importance. Each needs to be able to operate singly or with others, with guidance from the divine level. Kundalini flows more easily and is better assimilated when there is harmony among the bodies.

Control Exercise

Beginning with the physical body, ask to be in touch with each body in turn. Ask each body its opinion on which bodies may have too much control or input and which don't have enough. Ask each body how it feels about its role in the seven bodies. Write down any changes you feel would be appropriate to make.

Lie down, bring about a feeling that you are floating. Be aware of your divine level body. Ask it to be filled with God's Presence. Let the energy come into the soul level body and proceed down to each of the bodies, ending with the physical. Be in reflection for a few minutes.

The information given here on the seven bodies is brief, but it gives you enough to begin. For more information, refer to the The *Seven Bodies of Man in the Evolution of Consciousness*, and *The Seven Eyes of Man in the Evolution of Consciousness*.[1]

---

1. Both by the author, available by writing to Box 456, Melbourne, AR 72556.

Chapter 5

The Development of
the Four Brains

The transformation of the brains is one of the most noticeable changes caused by Kundalini cleansing. Genius, where extraordinary creative abilities and great moral and spiritual truths are available, is the ultimate state of the refined brain. In genius the brains receive and utilize information from universal and cosmic levels.

But the four brains are more resistant to Kundalini cleansing than any other areas because of aberrations in one's thinking and approach to life to which we are prone. Some, with excessive Kundalini that has not yet become useable, are left to vegetate in mental institutions; their problems are not understood.

Your skull actually changes shape, becoming larger during development of the brains. It may change shape a number of times, bringing searing headaches. Massaging the skull at the seams of the bones promotes expansion. Radiating excess Kundalini out around the head brings relief. Locate particularly sore spots on your scalp with your fingers; massage them to release the energy, letting your mind ramble, becoming aware of the thoughts or attitudes which prevented mind expansion. You may relive some tension by telling yourself it is okay to have the "big head."

Dr. Paul McClean has done some wonderful work with his Triune Brain Theory, very applicable to the seven body approach.

The Reptilian or First Brain
The first brain relates directly to the physical body and deals mainly with territorialism and survival. We all need to be comfortable with our territory or space, especially in Kundalini raising,

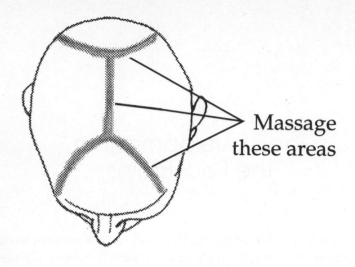

*Top of Skull—the jagged lines show where the skull bones come together.
Massaging in these areas reduces tension.*

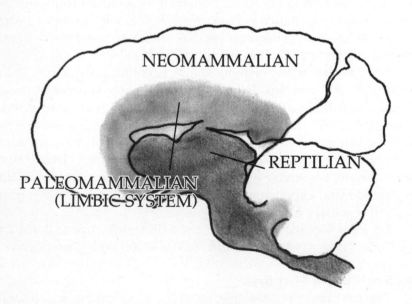

*The three levels of brains: (1) Reptilian—physical; (2) Limbic system—emotional;
(3) Neomammalian—mental.*

when we become over sensitive to others' energies and do not function as well in the world.

If you have had a poor sense of survival, you will notice an undercurrent of constant checking in yourself about the safety of places or situations. You will continually observe others either as threats or aids to survival. You will be overly concerned about "fitting in."

The Limbic System (Paleomammalian) or Second Brain

The second brain relates mainly to emotions and motivations and is connected with our emotional body. With an underdeveloped limbic system a person does not have good motivational skills, is not a good self-starter and will be excessively concerned about feelings.

The Third Brain (Neo-Mammalian)

The third brain incorporates both the left and right hemispheres. It relates to the mental body and is concerned with reason, logic, thinking, and creativity, acting much like a computer in that it works with information it has received through experiences and learning. The development of this brain is based partially on the healthy development of the first and second brains. With an underdeveloped third brain a person has difficulty using reason and logic to comprehend complex situations. He or she may be limited to one point of view and subject to rigidity or prejudice.

It has been said many times that we use approximately ten percent of our mental capacities. This may be due to underdeveloped first and second brains, inadequate stimulation, and laziness (defined as always taking the easy way, not using full perceptive and creative abilities). The result is that people think they are not in touch with all of their mental capabilities, that something is holding back their brain power.

When the first two brains are well developed, but the third not, a person will be overly concerned with feelings and territory; there will therefore be little interaction with others. In such a state a person may spend time with others, but not attentively (the attention is focused on the self). Of course, the same problems may occur when the first two brains are underdeveloped.

Excessively mentally developed people may display a lack of "good old common sense," as in "how can anyone so smart be so dumb?" Each brain has its own awareness, intelligence, and agenda, each its own concept of how the world functions and its relationship and position relative to these functions. Each brain may act either independently of or cooperatively with the other brains. Kundalini cleansing and refinement not only develops these brains but increases their interaction.

Children will not function well in school without good reptilian development; they tend either to be more combative and belligerent, or withdrawn. Children who lack a healthy sense of survival have low self-esteem. Their poorly developed limbic system may cause poor study habits, or they may be overly concerned with relationships.

The Fourth Brain

We live in a time of great mind expansion, not only involving increased development of three brains already mentioned but the development of a fourth brain. The new brain is still in the etheric (energy) stage; it has not yet manifested in the physical.

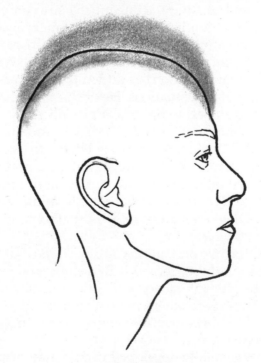

Area of etheric fourth brain.

Each brain overlaps the previous one (see illustration, opposite page). The first development of the fourth brain is under the crown chakra on top of the head, over the top of the two hemispheres of the third brain. It relates to the intuitional-compassionate level or fourth body and has a spiritual consciousness. Though it has not yet manifested in the physical, it is still useable. Where the main attribute of the third or mental brain is thinking, the main attribute of the fourth brain is awaring; a developed fourth brain will enable a person to receive new, previously unknown information. Tapping in the Universal Mind, the fourth brain will have limitless potential for receiving information.

There are etheric forms of brains five, six and seven, but their development is more distant. They relate to the corresponding bodies.

Exercises

For the Reptilian Brain

Meditate on how you feel about your territory; how can you change it to make it more supportive? Meditate on survival, to what extent it is an issue for you. What threatens or enhances your sense of survival?

Symbolism. Get a stuffed toy or picture of your favorite reptile. Feel connected to it occasionally during meditations.

Limbic System

Meditate on owning and enjoying your feelings. How many different feelings can you be aware at one time? Let cuddly feelings envelop your entire body; really enjoy them.

Symbolism. Color is highly related to and symbolic of emotions. To enhance and develop your emotions, make sure you have enough color in your life: in your surroundings, clothing, food, or artistic ventures.

Neo-Mammalian

Meditate on the left hemisphere, filling it with energy, then move the energy to the right hemisphere. Reverse the process and move energy from right to left hemisphere. Repeat this procedure several times. Feel the energy balance between the two sides and feel the *corpus collosum* (bridge between the two hemispheres) open for action. Give the entire area over to freedom and expansion.

Take some time each day to look hard at something; what else can you be aware of or see? This develops perception. Each day try to use your creativity. Read magazines or books on subjects you have not studied and in which you have no particular interest. This increases blood flow and helps open up new tracks in the brain; it also aids in expanding your ability to think and perceive.

Fourth Brain

Be aware of the area just below your crown chakra and across the top of your head under the skin. Move energy into this area, feeling it expand and open up.

Keeping your attention in the fourth brain area, ask questions, and let answers form. Don't rush the process; answers and pictures may take time to form. Meditate on using the information which comes to you through this awareness.

Kundalini Bath. Ask to feel and see the Kundalini energy as a golden light (mental); let it bathe inside your entire head, making sure each brain receives some attention. Vary the exercise by using a silvery light (spiritual). You may note heat in your head; this helps in the transformation, but when excessive brings headaches. For relief from headaches, equalize the energy throughout the head or send it out the crown chakra, mixing it with the divine energy above your head and letting the combination shower down around your body.

Chapter 6

Chakras

Introduction

Chakras are vortices through which energy flows both in and out the body. When developed, they rotate like a turning wheel. Most literature on chakras discusses seven main chakras, but we actually have hundreds, located all over the body. Each acupressure and acupuncture point is an energy vortex and therefore a chakra. The energy which powers these vortices comes from a number of sources, one being our own Kundalini or evolutionary energy, another being the spiritual force within us. These energies come from inside the body and flow out the chakras.

The chakras also receive. We may receive energy from other people, whether gently and imperceptibly or very aware of pulling it from them. When our energy is pulled by others, we may feel very sapped or "snagged" in a particular chakra. Being sent energy, we may feel bombarded. Spiritual energy, prana, and other energies all around us (we live in an ocean of energy), may also flow in through the chakra centers.

People less developed in their evolutionary growth tend to bring in much more energy than they give out. In weakness or illness, people may pull in energy from more vitalized or developed people. Those who feel weak, depleted or have a low self-image may be very strongly affected by others' energies, actually drawing on others, in which case they are called sappers. This name is unfair in some instances because the act of pulling energy from others may

53

make the difference in healing and getting enough strength to go ahead; it is a wonderful thing to be able to give energy to those who need it. Giving is part of our practice of visiting ill or depressed friends. We "give" energy from our chakras to theirs to help them.

Giving strengthens us; when energy is pulled or sucked from us, we can be weakened. There are people who habitually suck energy from others rather than develop their own; these may truly be called sappers. There is more information on this in Chapter 11.

People who are not very developed spiritually may be open to negative forces. Negative energy will come into their chakras, causing them to feel even worse than they do or to act in even more negative ways. A depressed person tends to put energies coming through the chakras on a depressed level, which only compounds problems.

Evolved people have more energy flowing out of their chakras than in. Their chakras look like flowers in bloom. As they become more highly developed, the Kundalini energy radiating from their chakras blends with divine energy, continues to radiate out, then

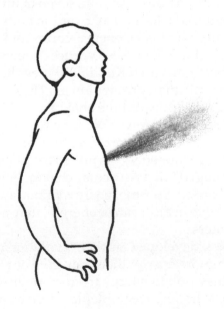

In a less developed chakra the energy flows directly out rather than rotating.

curves back to come in through the hands and feet (sometimes through other areas of the body), bringing a mixture of these energies into them.

Our growth and development are increasing during the Aquarian age; we go through many different moods and ways of being, relating to different chakras in the process. The chakras listed in this book help you gain a greater understanding of the different energy frequencies which control or affect our physical, emotional, mental, and spiritual states. During cleansing, you will find that fears or problems from this life and other lives may be locked or blocked at particular levels. You may also find joys or wonderful times which did not assimilate and were not released into the body cells, similarly blocked in the energy pattern. Sometimes fear of the future will be evident.

I suggest to beginning students of Kundalini that they let the energy flow directly out in front of their bodies rather than spin. Many times all of the petals are not fully developed and spinning only distorts the energy.

Kundalini Movement and Chakra Cleansing

There are many chakras in the body, but eight main ones will be used for this exercise, those in the areas of glands having extra importance in spiritual and evolutionary growth.

In the beginning, use the following chakras:
Navel
Solar Plexus
Heart (upper chest)
Throat (lower neck)
Fifth Eye (center of the forehead)
Crown Chakra (top of the head)

Do this exercise lying down or in the lotus position; take care that your back, neck and head are straight. It is much easier and generally safer to lie down. Place your attention on your lower back, above the tailbone area; DO NOT go as far down as the tailbone, as this may release extra Kundalini. Bring the energy from the lower back to the spine, then channel it out the front of the body through the navel chakra. Be aware of the energy flowing out. Do not force it.

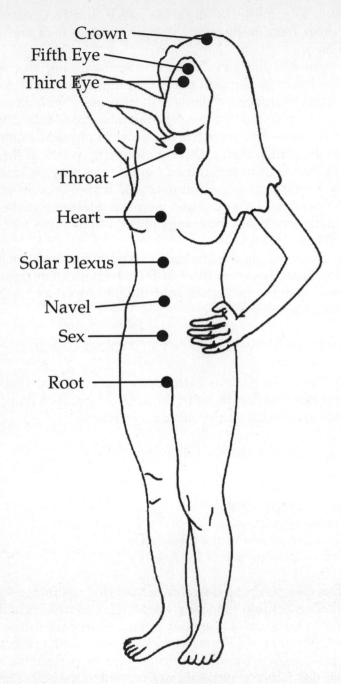

Crown

Fifth Eye

Third Eye

Throat

Heart

Solar Plexus

Navel

Sex

Root

Frontal Locations

Just let it happen. Be aware of the "feel" of the energy, the quality of the vibrations. You may experience strong feelings; if so, let them come. After a few minutes, bring the energy back to the spine, up and out the chakra in the solar plexus (just below the breast bone). Be aware of any change in the vibrational quality of the energies.

Continue bringing the energy back to the spine, up and out the next chakra. Always be aware of changes of vibrations, thoughts, feelings and whether an area seems blocked or overloaded; be aware, but do not get caught up in them. Just observe. If desired, make notes of your observations.

After sending the energy out the crown chakra, let the Kundalini energy (this is what is being directed) mix with the divine energy above your head (this divine energy is in the surrounding air at all times). Let this mixture shower over and penetrate into your body (see Chapter 15, Methods for Kundalini Release). Bathe your body inside and out with these beautiful energies from both polarities—heaven and earth—helping speed growth and development.

After you've done this exercise several times and become comfortable with it, add the sex chakra. When comfortable with that, add the root chakra (on the tailbone). *Note: We do not use the base chakra in this exercise because it may release too much energy.* When you start with the higher chakras, you clear a path so that if great amounts of energy are released in the sexual or root areas there is someplace for it to go; otherwise, the energy may become stuck and cause personality and health problems.

If there is pain or a problem near a chakra, omit that chakra from the exercise until the problem clears; the extra energy may make the situation worse.

Chakra Flows

An undeveloped person usually has numerous blocks around the edges of, or actually in, the chakras, slowing the energy or causing incorrect flow. After sufficient development and chakra cleansing I have students direct the energy in a circular motion such that it looks clockwise from the outside of the body, counterclockwise from inside the body. This movement puts the main force of the flow on the left, emphasizing the emotional and spiritual levels, establishing a more solid base to work from, and enhancing understanding of energies. At later stages I ask the students to reverse this flow;

this emphasizes the right side or mental level and develops psychic abilities, power, and force. The danger in developing the right side first is that students would not have the understanding and wisdom to use the energy well and may not only find themselves in a little more trouble but find many things happening to them they do not understand and do not know how to work with or control.

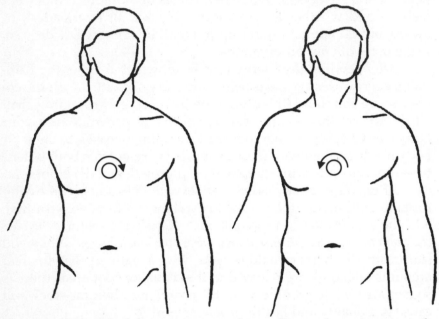

Note the rotating of the chakra energy goes over the top of the chakra to the left, bringing more of a feeling emphasis.

Same as Diagram 2 except over top to the right, with more of a mental emphasis.

In some people the general chakra flow is tipped upward; this generally indicates the Pollyanna type, who thinks everything is wonderful and sees only the good things in life. While it is nice to see the positive and the good, you must be aware of the negative side of people lest you get tripped up by them. The opposite situation is the person whose chakra flow is always headed toward the ground; such a person can be cynical, or in good times have great benevolence, though of a kind in which there is a feeling of condescension. When chakra flow tips more toward the right, a person will be judgmental and overly mental. When chakra flow tips to the left, a person may be overly emotional, trying to understand things to the point of not functioning well.

Chakras as observed from outside.

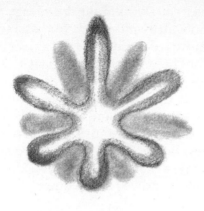

This flow indicates a pollyanna type person.

This flow indicates a cynical type person.

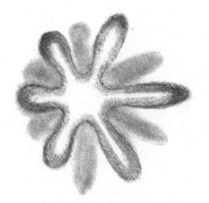

Right of body—The flow to the right of the body indicates an overly mental person.

Left of body—This flow to the left indicates an overly emotional person.

Some people have high amounts of poorly assimilated energy in the body such that the energy may flow in and out of the chakras with great force. When energy goes out in great force a person can be left manic or in states of unmaintainable ecstasy. The person does not have a good energy connection in the body. Energy drops and tends to go deep, creating a depressed state. The energy is literally pressed into the body. If you have these highs and lows, try not to let your highs be extremely high or your lows extremely low; work for balance. Try to feel the energy all over your body. Take the energy of the ecstasy or the depression, spread it all over the body and assimilate it into yourself until you feel more balanced.

In a more developed person, the chakras will gently flow in the direction which the person's destiny pattern requires. When needed, they will flow in the opposite direction. A chakra is much like a twirling bowl; in more developed people there will be smaller vortices flowing within this bowl, like petals just inside the rim. In the compassionate and loving heart chakra, for example, there are twelve petals. In the solar plexus chakra there are ten petals. There are twelve in the smaller crown chakra and 960 in the outer crown chakra.

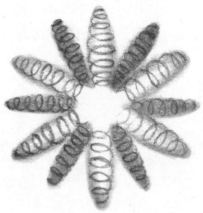

The lighter petals have energy flowing out while the darker petals indicate energy flowing in.

When a chakra and its petals flow correctly, a certain frequency is set up opening a person to psychic abilities or higher spiritual levels. A more highly developed person works at a higher octave of energy frequency. With a chakra cleansed and twirling correctly, a person has access through that frequency to higher octaves and may operate on higher dimensions. As psychic or spiritual abilities are developed, awareness and understanding of cosmic energy and other gifts abound.

Bear in mind that the beginner should not yet work for the higher octaves; until the areas are cleansed and properly aligned, distortions of energy, information and behavior may result, leaving a person feeling as if he or she had gone backwards in growth.

Don't get hung up on which symbol or color you are "supposed" to see in each chakra. As the chakras are cleansed and developed you will see many symbols, including the crescent moon, squares, stars, triangles, diamond shapes, and circles. Colors will change as you are working on various energies frequencies. Forcing yourself to work too early with the petals and the colors prescribed for each chakra (see chart # 1) can cause irritations and illness. As a person reaches to higher octaves (levels), the chakra colors will be brilliant or radiant. In an undeveloped state, the colors are very dull or dark areas may show.

Undeveloped people who have unbalanced chakra energy flow may relate to the world primarily through one or two chakras. Say one is a sexual chakra; it will not matter what you talk about, the person will soon turn it to a discussion of sex or use sexual terms. An overly emotional person will always get into feelings, no matter the

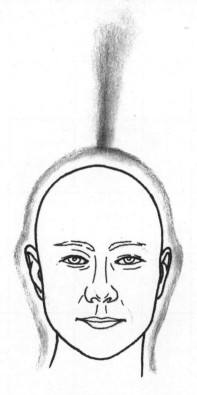

*The shadowy line indicates the location of the etheric
body on which the chakras are located.*

					Chart 1—CHAKRA	
Common Number	Sanskrit Name	English Name	Spinal Location	Frontal Location	Colors	Number of Petals
7	Sahasrara	crown	above 1st cervical	top of head	center-white and gold outer-chromatic	center-12 outer-960
		5th eye	above 2nd cervical	center of forehead	brilliant rainbow colors	16
6	Ajna	3rd eye	above 2nd cervical	between eyebrows	1/2 rose-yellow 1/2 blue-purple	96
5	Visudha	throat	above 3rd cervical	center of throat	silvery blue	16
4	Anahata	heart	above 5th thoracic	center of chest	green	12
		solar plexus	above 7th thoracic	solar plexus	yellow	24
3	Manipura	navel	above 10th thoracic	navel	orange	10
2	Svadhigh-thana	middle sex	above 1st lumbar	mid-point below navel	vermillion	6
1	Mudla-hara	root	coccyx		brilliant orange-red	4

INFORMATION				
Element	Powers	Glands Affected	Personality (P-positive)(N-negative)	Powers when Kundalini has activated astral Chakra levels
Spirit	speech	pineal	P-oneness with all, cosmic understanding N-put down feelings, alienated from life	able to leave body in full consciousness, greater understanding of life, perfections of astral functions
mind		pituitary	P-larger view of life N-narrow minded	akashic records
mind	cognition	pituitary	P-brotherhood, creative thinking N-wish to control others,egotistical	seeing of geometric shapes, colors, visions. Hear voice of higher self
ether	sounds	thyroid	P-reason, logic N-rigid,prejudiced, non-accepting views other than one's own	clairaudience, astral sounds, music
air	touch, feeling	thymus	P-compassion, intuitiveness N-hard hearted, closed, despairing	sensitive to the aches and pains of others—may find them in own body
	manifestation	pancreas	P-flexibility with energies—open to change and growth N-stuck, afraid to let new things manifest	senses coming changes and their appropriateness
fire	sight	leyden	P-peaceful, calm but colorful emotions N-over emotional, attached love	sensitive to astral influences, memory feelings, some memories of astral travel
water	taste	ovaries or testicles	P-vitality, sexuality N-lust, base emotions	basic understanding of cycles of creation/ destruction/birth/ death
earth	smell assimilation	adrenals	P-good self image, security through grounding with earth N-insecure, nothing to hold onto—out of touch with gravity	beginning of entry into the world of pure intelligence

subject. The overly mental may be unaware of the emotional and sometimes unaware of the body as well. We need, as much as possible, to work for balanced chakra flow.

The chakras are located in an etheric level just outside the body. As you develop this area you will find other chakras more distant from the body. On the outside edge of the emotional or astral aura, for example, there will be another chakra; outside the mental aura another, and so on through the seven bodies. These chakras eventually need to be developed, but their development is based on the development of the ones just outside of the physical body.

A radio has one basic energy coming into it—electricity. Changing the frequency of that energy makes it possible to receive different stations. It is similar with us; we have our basic Kundalini energy and spiritual energy and our chakras can change these energies to different frequencies. Some relate to emotions, some to sexual feelings or pure love, mental, psychic, healing abilities and various other functions. Learning to control and develop these areas is part of the training of mastering energies.

Chapter 7

The Chakras of the Seven Bodies

Introduction

As mentioned in Chapter 4, we have seven basic bodies or vibratory rates which our units of consciousness inhabit. Our chakras relate to these particular levels: physical, emotional or astral, mental, intuitional/compassionate, will/spirit, soul, and divine. The first three relate to our personality levels and the last four to our spiritual levels. Each of the seven bodies has seven different levels or sublevels, the vibratory rates of which correspond to the seven main bodies; for example, the physical body has sublevels of the physical, emotional or astral, mental, intuitional/compassionate, will/spirit, soul and divine. Each sublevel has its own energy vortices (chakras). The strongest chakras in each body are the double chakras—for example, the physical chakras of the physical body, the emotional centers of the emotional body, the mental level of the mental body. See Chart 1 in the previous chapter for information about the purpose of the chakras in relation to the body levels and sub levels. Chart 2 on the following page gives locations of all the sublevels.

All levels are interrelated; what affects one affects the others. A problem that manifests on a certain level in one body will also manifest on the corresponding level in the other six. For example, trouble at the emotional level in the physical body will mean trouble at the emotional level in the emotional, mental, intuitional/compassionate, will/spirit, soul and divine bodies. It is also true that release or

Chakras of the Planes→ / Chakras of the 7 Bodies↓	I Physical (Etheric) Chakras	II Emotional Plane (Astral) Chakras	III Mental Plane Chakras	IV Intuitional/ Compassionate Chakras	V Will/Spirit Chakras	VI Soul Level Chakras	VII Divine Level Chakras
Physical (Etheric) Body Chakras	Heels of feet & heels of hands	The spleen	Tops of shoulders & "sit bones" of pelvis	Slightly below cheekbones, inside jawbone	On breastbone in between the breasts	Adrenal glands above kidneys	Coccyx (Root chakra)
Emotional (Astral) Body Chakras	The stomach	Navel chakra (bellybutton)	Lower back, above root chakra & below small of back	Xiphoid process (Lower edge of breastbone)	Just below waist on spinal area of back	Approximately 2" to either side of compassionate heart chakra	Compassionate Heart chakra (center, upper chest)
Mental Body Chakras	Lower throat	The temples	Third eye, between eyebrows	Above navel, center of transverse colon	Upper throat at base of tongue, back under chin	The fifth eye (center of forehead)	Seventh eye, upper front of head (1/2-1" behind hairline)
Intuitional/ Compassionate Body Chakras	The liver	Outer Thighs, 1/2-way above knees & 1/2-way up upper arms	On breastbone, just above xiphoid process	Compassionate Heart Chakra	Both sides of nose, either side of nostrils	Pupils of the eyes	Medulla oblongatta, base of brain
Will/Spirit Body Chakras	Palms of hands & soles of feet	Backs of knees & insides of elbows	Armpits & "legpits"	1"-2" below the perineum (below the body)	Power/Sex chakra (approximately midway between navel & pubic bone)	Soft spot or 'Hole' in the back of head	This chakra is four fingers-width above the head
Soul Body Chakras	Instep of feet & thumb side of wrists (on bone)	Insides of legs just above knees & insides of arms just above elbows	Front edge of armpit & front where legs join pelvis	Ovaries or testicles	Approximately 1" above lower ribs, on either side of chest	Either side of neck, inside clavicle	Directly above ears on either side of head
Divine Body Chakras	Ends of fingers & ends of toes just under nails	Bone sticking out on back of head (devotional chakra)	Lower scallops of illium; pelvic bone	Solar plexus	"Horseshoe" at base of throat	Approximately 1-1/2" to left & to right of navel	Crown chakra (top center of head)

cleansing at one level will facilitate release or cleansing at its corresponding level in the other bodies. The ultimate goal is for all to be cleansed and in harmony, at which point we have our greatest power and sense of well-being.

Example. Trouble on the third (mental) level of the intuitional/compassionate body can cause a poor attitude toward the things you understand. It would appear either as a mindset that your understanding has no value, or as feeling that your understanding is absolute truth (making you inflexible and proud). This malfunction on the mental level of the intuitional/compassionate body will probably also cause a malfunction in your attitude toward your physical body, your feelings, your mental ability, and your power to think (will/spirit). When you have trouble accepting your physical body you may also have trouble at the physical level of every other body: your stomach (emotional body), throat (mental body), liver (intuitional/compassionate body), the palms and soles of your feet (will/spirit body), your instep and sides of the wrists (soul level body), and the ends of your toes and ends of the fingers (divine body).

Differences between the Piscean and Aquarian Ages

During the roughly 2600 years of the Piscean Age people have spent entire lives working primarily on one body or at the most two or three bodies; but now we need to cleanse and develop all bodies to achieve the necessary unity for utilizing the power of Aquarian Age energies. This is one reason so much unresolved karma seems to be coming to a head; we're experiencing a general housecleaning in all areas. People who have difficulty handling the powerful Aquarian Age cleansing energies may respond to the pressure of the energy and their inability to use it constructively by becoming angry, violent or depressed. Those who have already achieved good cleansing and unification in their bodies, or who are at least doing intensive cleansing work, will be able to use the Aquarian Age energies in constructive, joyful, creative, and spiritual ways.

One aspect of the Aquarian Age is increased awareness of the physical body and its functions. Most of us have been trained to rely primarily on our brainpower for information; but, tuning into the consciousness received through the body by the chakras, we will be more in tune with higher mental and spiritual energies and freer from restrictions and brain programming. Development and use of the brain was very important in the Piscean Age, but now we also need to expand to higher octaves of mental and spiritual energies.

Bodies and Chakras

The following diagrams show the locations of the seven chakra levels of each body. You may wish to be aware of troublesome areas in your own body and their corresponding chakras. In the next chapter you will find exercises to aid the cleansing and development.

Physical Body
The physical body is the densest of the seven bodies, the only one which can be seen without clairvoyant vision. Through the physical body we express, we receive, we become aware. These seven chakra levels comprise the physical body:

1. *Physical Level*
Four Locations: heels of the feet and hands.
Function: energy outlet for self assertion and for releasing physical aggressiveness; power spots.
Too open: very demanding.
Blocked: tendency to walk more on the toes; not to express the self or no desire to be noticed; a feeling of walking on egg shells; hands may seem cold and pulled back; difficulty in reaching out, shaking hands or touching others.

2. *Emotional Level*
Location: spleen.
Function: peace on the emotional level.
Too open: excessive anger expressed, sometimes in unhealthy ways.
Blocked: holding excessive anger which may be released in subconscious ways.

3. *Mental Level*
Four Locations: top of shoulders above the arm sockets and at the pelvic bone on either side (sit bones).
Function: expression of mental attitudes toward the body and its functioning in the physical world.

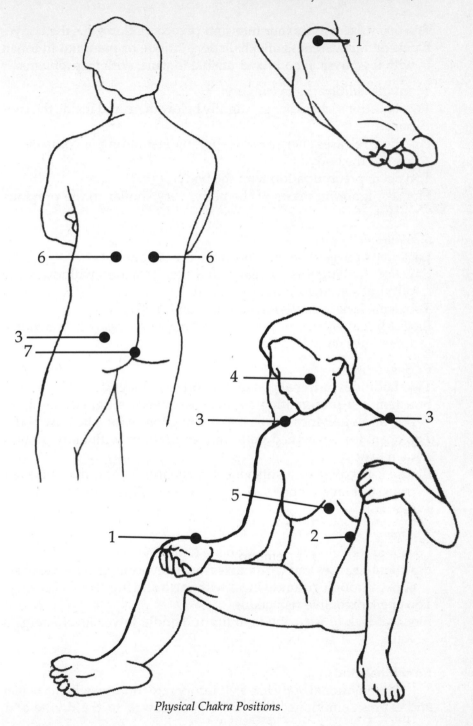

Physical Chakra Positions.

Too open: excessive awareness and preoccupation with the body.

Blocked: no awareness of exhaustion, fatigue or pain; not in touch with the physical body and unable to work with its problems.

4. *Intuitional/Compassionate Level*

Two Locations: cheekbones, slightly below them and inside the jaw-bone.

Function: releases energy for deeper understanding or compassion toward the body.

Too open: preoccupation with the body.

Blocked: ignoring needs of the body; very similar to the previous chakra.

5. *Will/Spirit Level*

Location: between the breasts on the breastbone.

Function: willingness to really live life; provides willpower for physical activities and for survival.

Too open: lack of caution when caution is needed.

Blocked: fear of really living or putting one's heart into actions; sometimes no will to live.

6. *Soul Level*

Two Locations: adrenal glands (on top of kidneys).

Function: self-preservation; awareness of need for fight or flight; action on an I AMness level; marshalling forces for a healthy body.

Too open: too concerned with fight or flight or with getting one's own way.

Blocked: needing to justify one's existence; feeling disconnected from soul level; repressed anger; open to illness and feelings of rejection.

7. *Divine Level*

Location: root chakra—coccyx bone (tail bone).

Function: cleanses and harmonizes lower level energies; sense of se-curity through groundedness with earth and higher level energy.

Too open: excessive risk taking.

Blocked: lack of security; inability to handle lower level energies well.

Emotional Body

The emotional body has a vibratory rate through which we feel and express emotions; it is also a passageway to the divine and when fully developed serves as an outlet for feelings of divine love.

1. Physical Level

Location: stomach.

Function: digestion of emotions.

Too open: gullible; excessive emphasis on feelings.

Blocked: inability to stomach or digest emotions; inability to act appropriately with emotions.

2. Emotional Level

Location: navel.

Function: strongest of the emotional chakras; connecting link with other people on feeling level.

Too open: too emotional; inability to think clearly because of the excessive pressure of the emotions.

Blocked: less refined or developed feelings; may be volcanic in nature; though energies may be blocked here a person would still be excessively preoccupied with feelings.

3. Mental Level

Location: in the lower back above the root chakra and below the small of the back.

Function: thinking or reasoning about feelings; humor and acceptance of life.

Too open: excessively preoccupied with feelings.

Blocked: no humor; taking feelings and self too seriously.

4. Intuitional/Compassionate Level

Location: xiphoid process (attached to bottom of breastbone).

Function: sorting out what is right or not right for the person; beginning of conscience energy.

Too open: excessive guilt feelings; always trying to justify or explain one's position or feelings.

Blocked: blocked guilt feelings; may take on others' expectations without understanding them.

5. Will/Spirit Level

Location: below the waist on the spine in the back.

Function: emotional strength; helps to balance emotions; aids in the feeling of having backbone.

Too open: pushing one's will on others through emotional means; excessively forceful.

Blocked: weak willed; easily swayed emotionally about others.

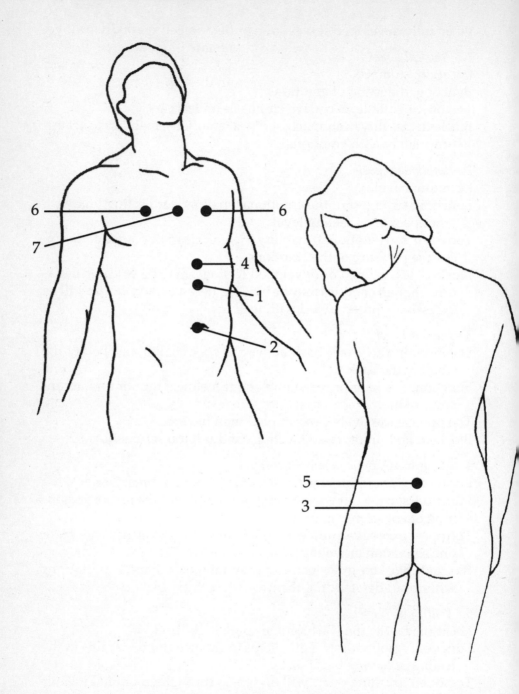

Emotional Chakra Positions.

6. Soul Level
Two Locations: both sides of compassionate heart chakra.
Function: helps strengthen your ability to give and receive love and to be aware of your own I AMness in the loving process.
Too open: may feel an excessive need to love others or be loved by others.
Blocked: not daring to love or not feeling worthy to love or be loved; blocks on the right side relate to attitudes about loving; blocks on the left side relate to feelings about loving.

7. Divine Level
Location: compassionate heart chakra (center of upper chest).
Function: feeling unity of all levels; integration of emotions for balance; equilibrium; love, compassion and understanding of others.
Too open: excessively concerned about loving enough; about doing enough for others; a person may feel wiped out.
Blocked: hard hearted; closed; afraid to love.

Mental Body
    The mental body is the vibratory rate through which we think and reason. When we operate in the lower levels of the mental body our thoughts and attitudes may be heavily influenced by feelings, giving rise to a "desire mind," products of which include prejudices, opinions, and other forms of emotionally-flavored thinking. Operating at the higher levels of the mental body we are capable of abstract thinking, creativity, logical reasoning, mathematics, and philosophy.

1. Physical Level
Location: lower throat.
Function: accepting what is; organizing ways to work with situations; a feeling of power to make changes.
Too open: always trying to take control of things, usually other people's lives.
Blocked: inability to accept (swallow) mentally; inability to work with situations; may have excessive pride or prejudices.

2. Emotional Level
Location: temples.
Function: feelings about things perceived.
Too open: excessive attempts to comprehend everything.

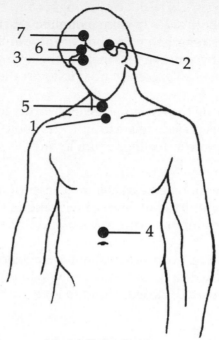

Mental Chakra Positions

Blocked: may distort vision or only see what is comfortably perceived.

3. *Mental Level*
Location: third eye (between eyebrows).
Function: home of ego; strengthens self as separate individual; psychic sight.
Too open: egotistical.
Blocked: weak or reversed ego; closed to other dimensions of life.

4. *Intuitional/Compassionate Level*
Location: center of transverse colon (above navel).
Function: emotional level of acceptance or rejection of thoughts; emotional-mental connection.
Too open: feeling one's thoughts are excessively important.
Blocked: undigested thought forms or ideas; can lead to constipation.

5. *Will/Spirit Level*
Location: upper throat, at the base of the tongue and straight back under the chin.

Function: activates will to express thoughts and speak up.

Too open: excessive expression of thoughts (talk too much).

Blocked: lack of confidence in one's mental abilities; choking on words; sore throat.

6. Soul Level

Location: fifth eye (center of forehead).

Function: activates higher mind for creative thinking; brings awareness of the larger picture of life and one's place in it.

Too open: too preoccupied with altruistic values.

Blocked: self-centered; lack of vision.

7. Divine Level

Location: seventh eye (straight up from the fifth eye, above the normal hair line about $3/4$ to 1 inch).

Function: awareness of self on soul level; communication point with higher self.

Too open: excessively preoccupied with higher vision of the self.

Blocked: inability to perceive and use spiritual insights; preoccupied with just the human side of life.

Intuitional/Compassionate Body

This is the vibratory rate where one feels compassion and has understanding of self and others. It is also a vehicle for the expression of higher forms of love—a gateway to the Divine—serving as a connecting link between the emotional and the divine levels. In this body, we are above the limits of time and space; there is understanding without the need to go through a process of reasoning and thinking. This body is the home of intuition.

1. Physical Level

Location: liver.

Function: energy for acting on what you spiritually believe is correct for you.

Too open: unawareness of how your spiritual direction can best work with other people's spiritual direction; too pushy with your insights.

Blocked: lily-livered; may feel like a coward in terms of following through on your own spiritual understanding.

2. Emotional Level

Four Locations: midpoint on outer edges of thighs and upper arms.

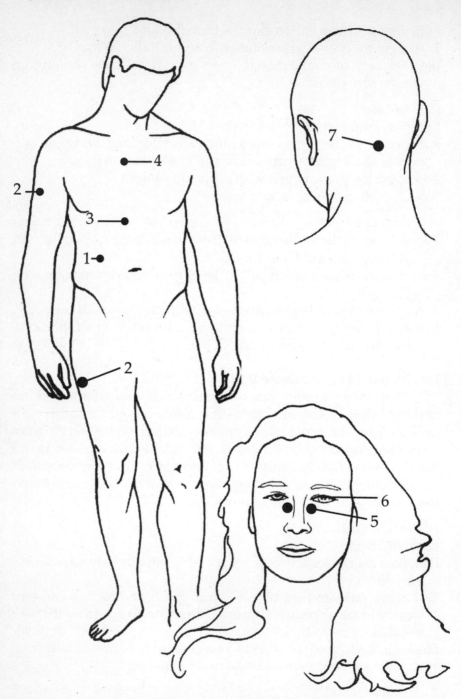

Intuitional/Compassionate Chakra Positions.

Function: connection with other people; feeling the flow of energy between you and others.

Too open: overly aware of other people's energy and not balancing with your own.

Blocked: shut off from others.

3. *Mental Level*

Location: bottom part of the breastbone above the xiphoid process.

Function: flowing appropriately in life and relationships.

Too open: over acceptance.

Blocked: too attached or rejecting.

4. *Intuitional/Compassionate Level*

Location: heart chakra—upper center of chest (this chakra is the same as the seventh level of the emotional body).

Function: most important of all chakras for expressing unconditional love, compassion and understanding.

Too open: overly concerned with others; lack of balance between self and others.

Blocked: hard-hearted; conditional love, compassion and understanding.

5. *Will/Spirit Level*

Two Locations: both sides of upper nose.

Function: power chakras, providing courage to combine energy of earth and heaven for practical use.

Too open: excessive either with earth or heavenly energies; inability to bring energies back into the self.

Blocked: feel powerless or ineffectual in the above areas.

6. *Soul Level*

Two Locations: pupils.

Function: deep expression of the I AMness presence; sometimes called windows to the soul.

Too open: excessive need to feel profound.

Blocked: afraid of one's own profoundness; the eyes may look as if there is nobody in there (may feel this when looking at people).

7. *Divine Level*

Location: base of brain, medulla oblongata.

Function: stimulates divine understanding; bliss awareness of self as one with God; harmonizes understandings from insights on lower levels and of the divine plan in one's life.

Too open: preoccupied with higher levels at the expense of the human level.

Blocked: preoccupied with the human level and the mundane awareness of life.

Will/Spirit Body

The will/spirit body is the vehicle or vibratory rate through which spirit expresses. It channels energy which manifests as will and is the highest level a person can reach and still negate the Divine or Soul levels; this brings a possibility of great negativity or karma because the energy is so high that it can cause, when misused, much destruction. This is the area for choice—Divine will or the individual will.

1. *Physical Level*

Four Locations: palms of hands and soles of feet.

Function: feeling energy in relationship to outside world.

Too open: too involved with others; excessive wishing to share or fix the world.

Blocked: poor circulation; cold in hands or feet; holding back from sharing with the world.

2. *Emotional Level*

Four Locations: backs of knees and insides of elbows.

Function: ability to assert oneself on the emotional level and be open to action from the feeling level.

Too open: too assertive.

Blocked: weak knees; lack of emotional support for one's will or desires.

3. *Mental Level*

Four Locations: armpits and area where legs connect with the body on the front side.

Function: mental acceptance of one's will and desires; putting thinking into action.

Too open: too egotistical.

Blocked: poor attitude toward self; fear and holding back in areas.

4. *Intuitional/Compassionate Level*

Location: one inch below the crotch.

Function: provides energy for understanding and use of power; companion chakra to the seventh level chakra of this body.

Too open: caution should be used with this chakra; the power can be negative when your body is not developed to handle higher energies.

Blocked: intensifies negative sexual energies; increases feelings of violence or a need to explode.

5. *Will/Spirit Level*

Location: power sex chakra (two chakras below navel).

Function: power source for physical energy, sex drive, healing energy, joy of life.

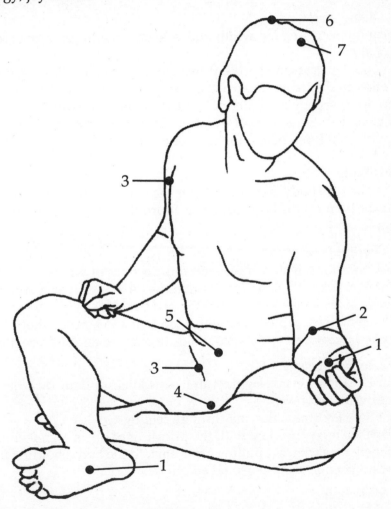

Will/Spirit Chakra Positions.

Too open: excessive or uncontrolled power or sexual energy.

Blocked: fear of power, lack of joy, negative or perverse sexual energy.

6. *Soul Level*

Location: behind crown chakra at top of head.

Function: aids in reaching nirvana or bliss states; it is the "not my will, but thine" chakra.

Too open: spaced out, inability to use higher energies in daily life.

Blocked: clouds awareness of higher spiritual and mental levels.

7. *Divine Level*

Location: four fingers' width above head, smaller than the crown chakra.

Function: human and spiritual energies blend here, allowing one to enter higher levels in an active, practical way.

Too open: spacey or depleting of physical body energy.

Blocked: brings feelings of isolation, loneliness, lack of connection with soul level, being down on oneself.

Soul Body

The soul body is the vehicle for the expression of soul energies and the home of the I AM presence. It provides guidance for the human level.

1. *Physical Level*

Four Locations: instep of feet and thumb sides of wrists.

Function: strengthens ability to bring the I AMness presence into action; gives soul expression in the physical level.

Too open: preoccupied with self; a tendency to ignore others.

Blocked: weak feet and hands; holding back generally from life.

2. *Emotional Level*

Four Locations: inside legs just above the knees and inside arms just above the elbows.

Function: I AMness flowing through feelings.

Too open: too concerned with the priorities of one's own feelings.

Blocked: weak-kneed; pulling arms back to the body; holding back from deeper, more personal emotions.

3. *Mental Level*

Four Locations: inside connections of legs with pelvic area and on the body side of the armpits.

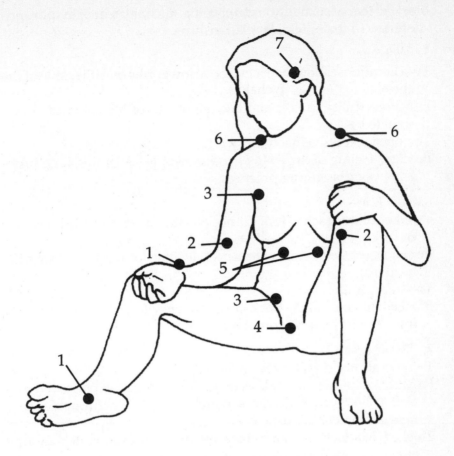

Soul Chakra Positions.

Function: I AMness expressed through mental reasoning; a logical
  or healthy attitude toward self as a person and unit.
Too open: preoccupied with expressing self as a person or unit.
Blocked: poor posture; not feeling justified in life; disconnected between mental and soul areas.

4. Intuitional/Compassionate Level

Two Locations: ovaries or testicles.
Function: development of sexual orientation toward self and the
  world; healthy polarity identities.
Too open: feeling that one is God's gift to the opposite sex.

Blocked: fear of sexuality and not being spiritual; fear of inappropriateness in male/female relationships.

5. *Will/Spirit Level*

Two Locations: about one inch above lower ribs on either side of the chest.

Function: ability to take and use the breath of life; asserting one's right to be.

Too open: excessive need for space.

Blocked: feeling of drowning in other people's energies; lung problems; poor breathing practices.

6. *Soul Level*

Two Locations: each side of the neck on the curve from the body into the neck.

Function: expression of self-respect; feelings of worth; holding the head up.

Too open: pride.

Blocked: tension in the neck area; tendency to pull neck and head into the body (turtle complex).

7. *Divine Level*

Two Locations: directly above the ears.

Function: experiencing self as one with God; self experienced as a unit of God's consciousness; directing one's life through awareness of God consciousness.

Blocked: headaches; poor perception or insight as to one's destiny energies; a feeling of "losing it."

Divine Body

The Divine body is the seventh and the highest. In this body we relate to the spark of the divine within us. Through this energy we can deeply feel the presence of God in our lives and feel oneness with God (you may wish to use the term divine reality, source— whatever describes this energy for you).

1. *Physical Level*

Twenty Locations: ends of fingers and toes.

Function: healing energies and perceptions of energies around you.

Too open: drains energy.

Blocked: may turn into anger and a desire to push or kick one's way clear, symbolically or literally; can affect health of hands and feet.

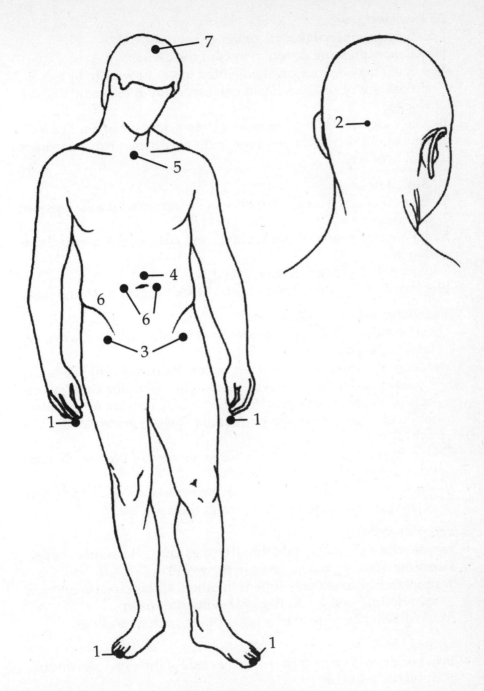

Divine Chakra Positions.

2. Emotional Level

Location: devotional chakra, center of back of head.

Function: expressing devotion toward the divine.

Too open: may be excessively devoted to your own ego or a cause (fanaticism or over-zealousness), especially if the crown is also blocked.

Blocked: lack of feeling, interest or even acknowledgment of a divine level or beings or one's connection with this area; sometimes cold to others.

3. Mental Level

Two Locations: just inside the pelvic bones above where the legs join the body.

Function: expression of thankfulness and faith; opens one to abundance.

Too open: Pollyanna behavior; greedy.

Blocked: may limit thankfulness and block the flow of abundance.

4. Intuitional/Compassionate Level

Location: solar plexus, just below the xiphoid process chakra; relates to the pancreas.

Function: spiritual energies enter in for distribution to the body; awakens and refines the system to higher vibrations and sweetness of life; many energies flow through this chakra for manifestation of circumstances in one's life; relates to one's place in the world.

Too open: searching excessively for sweetness of life; overly concerned about one's place in life.

Blocked: closed to spiritual energies, sweetness and joy of life; fear of change and opening up to greater things in life.

5. Will/Spirit Level

Location: in hollow at base of throat (bones form a horseshoe shape).

Function: desire or will to serve in the world.

Too open: excessive commitment to others at the expense of one's own destiny-energy; feelings of saving the world.

Blocked: fear of giving to or serving others; martyr feelings.

6. Soul Level

Two Locations: 1, to 1+ inches on either side of the navel (depending upon body size).

Function: unification of the energies of the body with divine energies or with others.

Too open: excessive search for oneness.

Blocked: can be destructive to self or others.

7. *Divine Level*

Location: crown chakra, center of top of head.

Function: connection with higher spiritual levels; balance in everyday life.

Too open: spacy; unable to function in daily life; may feel drained or
weak.

Blocked: negativity; down on oneself; lack of connection with divine levels; unbalanced; confusion.

Chapter 8

Development of
the Chakras

How to Work with Chakras

It is best to work with only one level of one body of chakras at a time. The most effective procedure is to begin at the physical level of the physical body; proceed to the emotional of the physical, the mental, et cetera, continuing until you have finished all seven levels of the physical body. Having completed work on the physical body, move on to the emotional, mental, and so on through all the bodies.

Make an exception to this rule if a particular chakra or body is painful, very tight, or is trying to open on its own, in which case you may wish to begin with that location. Complete all of the chakras on that body; then start with the physical and work upwards.

It is best to work on only one body at a time because you may become too buzzed, spacey or confused doing too many bodies at once.

Cleansing and Opening Chakras

1/ With your hand, find the location of the chakra or chakras on your body. Follow the directions, looking at the areas shown in the picture in the previous chapters. Generally, the energy of the chakras will feel different from that of the surrounding areas.

2/ Massage the chakra lightly. This helps open it and release any blocks. If there is much pain, do not massage; instead, hold your hand over the chakra and send energy into it. The extra energy helps release the block. Further assist release by imagining the energy going from your hand into the chakra; energy follows imagination. After a few moments release the chakra. Do not press hard on the xiphoid process, as it can be damaged easily.

3/ Either lie down or sit comfortably. Let go completely and let thoughts or feelings come to you. When energy is released from a chakra, information comes to your awareness; it may be a strong message, a memory of an incident, or an attitude. Let your mind ramble. The time necessary for these messages to come through varies from a few moments to as much as fifteen or thirty minutes. Do what feels comfortable to you, but do not stop the process too soon. If nothing comes and you feel comfortable with letting it go, fine; but if you feel restless, uncomfortable or irritable you probably should continue. Remember, the blocks may have existed for a long time and you may not wish to reblock or hold things back. When cleansing is completed, you will generally experience a release of energy and feel refreshed and energized.

Energy Flows

At the start, try to let the energy come straight out of your chakras, refraining from spinning the chakras in either direction. Simply let the energy come out in a direct manner until the area feels free and clear. If you wish, in later work, you may spin your chakras so that the energy going over the top of the chakra goes to the left side (clockwise from the outside). As long as the energy flows or spirals away from the body you will be at a refined emotional or spiritual level. But if the energy spirals back into the body it can cause negative or depressing feelings. Sometimes you may wish to spiral energy over the top of the chakra to the right side of the body (counterclockwise from the outside), putting you in touch with the mental or high mental vibrations for as long as the energy radiates away from the body (spiraling back into the body it will again cause depressive attitudes and negative perceptions).

Experiment with the flow of your chakras. In the beginning it will be difficult to be aware of direction, but with practice you will develop greater awareness and more control over your life.

Posture

People commonly sit or stand in a manner that blocks good chakra flow. You may, for instance, have trouble dealing with your

I-AMness and feeling good about yourself, in which case you may round your shoulders or bend your body to close off level three of the soul level body, or tighten your elbows and knees to block off those feelings. Another possibility is that you may curve in your chest as a way of blocking off the various chakras on the breastbone and compromise your will to live (level five of the physical body). Watch your posture. If you feel that by the way you carry yourself you block chakras, work on those particular chakras to find out what thoughts or feelings they contain; you could gain much insight into your attitude toward yourself.

Awareness

Awareness of posture change, aches, pains, or tensions can all be little signs that something is going wrong with the energy pattern some place in the body. It is always the chakras of those areas that will be affected. We ourselves can close them off subconsciously through fear, turning away from things, or holding back. Doing so, we pull the energy into the body, causing heaviness, depression, or blocked muscles.

When we feel light and joyful, the energy flows out, radiating from our bodies and opening our chakras. During a particularly joyous, happy, up-time, energy in blocked areas tends to release; thus several days later you may find yourself depressed, down, and in need of dealing with the released energy. But if you go with it, work with it, and allow it to continue the cleansing, it should not be long until you are feeling very, very good again.

Recommendations

I recommend developing the fifth eye before working with the third eye, as anything the third eye can do the fifth eye can do better. The danger in working intensely with the third eye first is that it is so connected with ego it may foster spiritual pride. The fifth eye helps develop the bigger picture beyond the individual picture. I also recommend developing the "will to live" heart chakra first in order to enhance heart strength. Developing the compassionate heart chakra first may lead to becoming overly compassionate and drained; it is not good to give too much from a heart chakra until the power is built from within and one learns to channel energy through it.

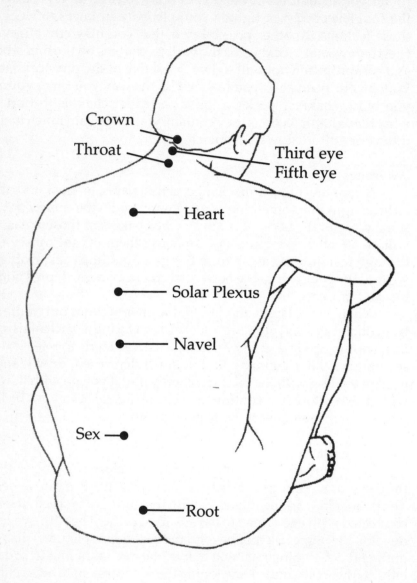

Chakra Openings on the Spine

Front Chakras versus Back Chakras

This book is primarily concerned with the spinal chakras opening in the front rather than in the back. Unless the front areas are cleaned and vitalized, energy from the spine will be blocked; as the front chakras open, the nadis or connections from the front chakras to the spinal openings automatically open. In addition, working on the spinal openings may bring an excessive interest in phenomena harmful to a person's growth, interesting perhaps, but not of primary importance in growth.

Opening up Body Energy

Stand in the middle of the room. Get the feeling of letting your energy go out from your whole body to fill the entire room, even the corners. This is a method of releasing energy from and balancing the chakras (including those not listed in this book). Doing this strengthens your aura. You can hold back other people's energies and may then become aware from the outer edge of your aura how others feel or think, as opposed to having the energy come in and affect your body. In addition, as your aura is strengthened, your outgoing energies are tempered and modified by the general energy in your aura and will not affect others as heavily.

Sending and Receiving Energy

Chakras are energy transmitting and receiving stations. We transmit energy, turning it into messages or feelings for other people. But we are constantly receiving from others, sometimes subliminally or subconsciously and at other times in a very aware state. More often than not the energy of others is an intrusion on our own energy patterns and may leave us thinking we have moods, thoughts, or feelings to work out which are not actually our own; or the intruding energies may just slow us down. We may also think we have an illness, pain, or tension.

Exercise

Exercise is very important in helping to even out the energy moving through the body. Many problems work themselves out just through physical exercises. Yoga is a particularly good form of exercise to maintain better chakra condition. Free form dance is also helpful; as you dance you emphasize different movements of your body, releasing blocked energy. Rest is also very important, allowing your system to balance energies and make its own adjustments; often if you just leave your body alone for a while, let it rest, it does much to heal itself and release blocked areas.

Opening and Developing the Chakras of the Seven Bodies

The following is a series of meditative exercises to be used in opening and developing the chakras described in Chapter 7. It may be done alone or with other people.

If a particular chakra area hurts, don't massage it; just send energy into it, either mentally or from the ends of your fingers, breaking down the energy form creating the pain. The body sends a subtle communication. In touch with it, you will sense what to do and what not to do. But even when you listen, if your body resorts to pain and you don't deal with that area, the energy may cause disease or illness. If the energy is too congealed, too blocked, or too constipated, you can attract accidents that release it. Much exhaustion and pain may occur in the physical chakras. Your body has a strong sense of self-healing; given proper time and tools, it will come around. Astrological energies, diet, overwork or general inattentiveness to your body also influence your physical well being.

Bodies are living machines. As with any living machine, there are knobs to pull or buttons to push. The chakras are the buttons and knobs of the human machine. Our way of living and relating to life is affected very heavily by chakra flow. Through the release of energy these exercises produce, you will become aware how really important your chakras are in life, understanding in the process how you block yourself from life and consciousness, how you enhance the present, or how, just by chakra flow, you open yourself to new things. As you tune into the chakras, let your consciousness be with them and let the energy or consciousness of the chakra answer you.

The Physical Body

1. Physical Body-Physical Level: Heels of feet.
Stand in an area where you have plenty of room to walk around. Feel energy in your heels. Begin breathing through your

hands, through your feet and through the top of your head. Be very aware of the heels. Continue to walk around, feeling energy in your feet. Walk firmly with your heels, really asserting yourself. Feel the energy flow. Many people stop the energy at their ankles, which causes foot trouble. If you wish, sit or lie down and enter a meditative state; let information come to you about your heels: your assertiveness, your willingness to make your mark in the world.

Physical Body-Physical Level: Heels of hands.

Many people do not really get their hands into handshakes. Their fingers tentatively reach out and the strength of their hand is not there. Do you shake hands with your fingers? Or do you get the whole hand in there, so that the heel of your hand touches the other person's hand? Be aware of that part of your hand and how much can you get it into action. Doing this exercise with others, take turns shaking hands. How does it feel to have full handshakes?

2. *Physical Body-Emotional Level: Spleen.*

Relax the spleen. Ask it if you are still holding any anger from your childhood; if you find some, spread it all over your body, thus diffusing it (defusing, too), making it easier to learn from and manage. As the anger moves around your body, turn it into strength and understanding.

The spleen functions in part as a safety valve for overloaded emotions. Put your awareness in the spleen area and ask about any emotional overload; finding some, work on a healthy understanding and release situations. When you cannot work them out yourself, find a therapist to help you.

3. *Physical Body-Mental Level: Tops of the shoulders (in the "V" area between the top of the shoulder bones) and the part of the pelvic bone used for sitting.*

This level concerns mental attitudes you have toward your body. Massage the tops of the shoulders; really let them relax. Ask the chakras if there is some exhaustion or pain from the past that you have blocked. Sometimes we can be tired from old pain. If you find it, release the energy through your system and acknowledge it. As you let it go, turn the tiredness or physical pain energy into strength. If you feel like lead and aren't moving well, it may be due to these chakras. You can let the energy flow out in a very positive, beautiful way and feel good about your physical body.

4. *Physical Body-Intuitional/Compassionate Level: Slightly below the cheekbones and near the jawbone.*

Massage these areas well; if you want to wake them more, send energy into the chakras. Tune into the chakras and ask what they have to say about your body. You may feel your entire body relax.

5. *Physical Body-Will/Spirit Level: Between the breasts and the breastbone.*

Ask what areas of life you really put your heart into; where do you have the will to live? Then ask where you lack the will to live or where you hold back.

6. *Physical Body-Soul Level: Adrenal glands, on top of the kidneys in the back.*

These may be called flight or fight chakras, giving you, as necessary, the energy to fight or to get away. They relate to self-preservation and healing. It is possible to repress so much anger in them (literally depressing the energies) that your adrenalin can no longer flow; of course this can lead to depression. Talk to your adrenal glands; ask where you should fight a little harder and where you should let go. Then ask what illness ensues from repressing your energies there.

7. *Physical Body-Divine Level: Root chakra on the tailbone.*

This level can bring a sense of security. Ask the chakra what adds to your security and what gives you a sense of insecurity and needs to be taken away. This level can also cleanse and harmonize your lower level energies.End the exercise of the physical body chakras by stretching all over. You may also wish to listen to music or dance to music as a way of vitalizing the energy and helping it flow. Send love and appreciation to your body.

Emotional Body

1. *Emotional Body-Physical Level: Stomach.*

This chakra relates to your ability to stomach things or digest what happens to you, not just on the physical level but with your emotions. Lightly massage your stomach; relax it. Be in touch with your stomach and ask what emotions you need to digest better.

2. *Emotional Body-Emotional Level: The navel.*

This is the main location of our emotions and feelings. As you tune into this chakra, ask for positive, beautiful feelings that you should express more. Then ask the chakra what negative or volcanic feelings are stored there.

3. Emotional Body-Mental Level: Lower back on the spine just above the root chakra.

This chakra relates to your attitude about your feelings. Are you overly serious? Do you have a sense of humor with them? Massage the chakra and ask where in life you take yourself too seriously; ask also what you need to take more seriously.

4. Emotional Body-Intuitional/Compassionate Level: The xiphoid process, on the end of the breastbone.

In its deeper sense this chakra relates to inner direction—the still, small voice within. In its more negative sense it may relate to guilt feelings and restrictions imposed by others. Lightly massage it. Ask if you have guilt feelings that have been implanted from others. Go deeper; ask what guilt feelings you have heard from your own still, small voice. Meditate and work on any you find. This area also relates to profoundness and a deep sense of who you are and how you are to develop; it is like the seed of the self. Ask this chakra how you can be truer to your self.

5. Emotional Body-Will/Spirit Level: Below the waist on the spine.

This chakra represents an emotional will bringing strength to your feelings. Not used well, it reverses and makes you overly emotional. Massage the area and ask in what areas you need to have more positive strength from your feelings and in what areas you get too emotional.

6. Emotional Body-Soul Level: Chakras on both sides of the compassionate heart chakra.

The chakra on the left relates to your feelings about loving. Do you feel good about it? Does loving make you happy or do you feel guilty for loving? The chakra on the right side is related to mental attitudes—"I should be loving this person," or "I shouldn't be loving this person"—and feelings of having the right to love. If your compassionate heart chakra is flowing and open you know the ones on either side of it are clear.

These chakras put conditions on your love. Massage them both; let the energy flow. Ask the left one how it puts conditions on your loving; then ask the one on the right where it puts conditions on your loving. Get the feeling of their openness. Allow the compassionate heart chakra between them to relax (see next chakra).

7. Emotional Body-Divine Level: Center of upper chest.

Massage this area; let it open up. Think of the companion chakras as relaxed and open. Do you feel secure enough within yourself to let energy flow from here in unconditional love to other people? This doesn't mean you have to like or approve of the others' thoughts or actions, only that you can love unconditionally. Ask the chakra whom you do and do not love unconditionally.

Mental Body

1. Mental Body-Physical Level: Lower throat just above the horseshoe.

This chakra is very important because it concerns accepting what is and organizing ways to work with it. It can release much power. Accepting does not mean you have to like it or put up with it, rather that you acknowledge and accept that something is the way it is; you then gain the power to organize and do something with it.

Take deep, peaceful breaths. Open yourself in that chakra as much as possible. Ask what two areas in life you need to accept and work with more. Also ask for ideas on how to do this. Ask for two areas in which you are doing very well and can quit hassling yourself about.

2. Mental Body-Emotional Level: The temples.

This area concerns how you feel about what you see. You may tense up and cause distortion in your vision so you see only what you want to or what you think you can handle. Massage the temples. Let the energy flow and ask the consciousness of the temples what it has blocked because you don't want to see it. Ask what you can do to see things with more clarity and depth.

3. Mental Body-Mental Level: Third eye between the eyebrows.

This eye is connected with the ego and energizes a sense of the human self. Ask this eye in what area you let too much ego fog your vision; also ask where you are doing well.

4. Mental Body-Intuitional/Compassionate Level: The center of the transverse colon about midway between the navel and solar plexus chakra.

This chakra concerns understanding your thoughts. Do you think you have the right attitudes in life? This may be another "hassle" chakra; due to unintegrated thought forms or unassimilated ideas, it may lead to constipation. Send some energy to the chakra to open it up and ask to know three areas of life in which you need to be more compassionate toward your own thoughts and ideas.

5. *Mental Body-Will/Spirit Level: Upper throat, straight back under the chin and under the base of the tongue.*

This chakra concerns expression of thought and speaking up. Blocked, it may cause a lack of confidence in mental abilities, choking on words, a sore throat, loss of clarity or freedom in speech. Massage the chakra. What areas of life are difficult to discuss for you? What areas are open?

6. *Mental Body-Soul Level: Fifth eye (center of forehead).*

The soul level of the mental body activates the higher mind and allows you to see the bigger picture. Without sufficient openness in it you will not even comprehend that there are areas of knowledge beyond your knowing. When this chakra is closed, you may feel as if you know it all but be very unaware. Massage the fifth eye. Let energy flow out. Ask where you are doing well to expand your comprehension of the bigger picture and where you are holding back.

7. *Mental Body/Divine Level: Seventh eye (about $3/4$-1 inch above the normal hairline or about 1-1$^1/_4$ inch from the sixth eye.*

Moving your finger lightly in this area, you may feel the chakra. Massage it and ask to see a white light from the spiritual level. If light comes in a muddy or dark color instead, you know that you either need to develop this chakra more or go through more cleansing. If you don't see the light at all you still might be aware of its coming into the system. Let the white light from the seventh eye (whether you see it or feel it) come down and go out the third eye to cleanse and uplift the ego; then feel those energies all over your body.

Intuitional/Compassionate Body

1. *Intuitional/Compassionate Body-Physical Level: The liver, located on the right side of the body with some under the rib cage and some extending below.*

This chakra concerns acting on what you believe is spiritually right for you. Lightly massage the area. If there is any pain there, do not massage but just let energy release. Then ask to know a time when you acted on what you spiritually believed was correct for you. How did it feel? Then ask to remember some times when you felt "lily-livered" and you did not follow through.

2. Intuitional/Compassionate Body-Emotional Level: Midpoint on the outside edges of the thighs and upper arms.

These chakras concern relating to other people. Relax your upper arms and massage the chakras. Relax your thighs and massage the chakras there. Visualize the different people with whom you have relationships. Thinking of each one, do these chakras want to open or close? Because we are called upon in the New Age to be deeper and closer friends with many people, it is important to be able to relax these chakras. Practice when you are with people in whose company you habitually tighten these chakras.

3. Intuitional/Compassionate Body-Mental Level: The bottom of the breastbone just above the xiphoid process.

This chakra has much to do with whether you flow with life, reject life or become excessively attached. Energy in this chakra that becomes twisted may produce a very cynical or sharp tongue and generally make you difficult to get along with; there may be humor, but it is often so sharp that others feel cut to shreds. Massage the chakra; let it flow. Ask where you are too attached and where you are too rejecting. Then ask to know where you are doing well.

4. Intuitional/Compassionate Body-Intuitional/Compassionate Level: Between the breasts, halfway between the horseshoe and the chakras.

When this chakra is too open you may find you are overly compassionate and you are draining yourself. It is also possible to close this chakra and become hard-hearted. Remember, this is the same chakra as the divine level of the emotional body; it is incredibly important. Through it we feel unconditional love and compassion; our intuitions function at a high level, lifting our life to a much more spiritual level. Massage the chakra. Does it feel tight, or too open? Let the energy flow and ask the chakra in what situations you are too compassionate and in what you are too hard-hearted.

5. Intuitional/Compassionate Body-Will/Spirit Level: On either side of the nose.

These are the power chakras. I sometimes call them "Native American chakras" because they concern combining the power of heaven and the power of earth to bring courage and understanding into daily life. Massage them. You may wish to ask if you have a strong Native American past life during which these chakras were very open and well used. Then ask in what situations in this life you need more openness in these chakras. When do you block them?

6. *Intuitional/Compassionate Body-Soul Level: Pupils.*

It is through these chakras that you can most truly see into another's soul and others can see into yours. If you are alone, you may wish to look in a mirror; see how deeply you can look into yourself. If you are with others, look deeply into their eyes and let them look deeply into yours. Are you embarrassed or uncomfortable, as though you were being totally bared? Many people have difficulty in truly being open from this level. To make things easier, you may wish to do this exercise looking softly. Keeping energy in your back may give you strength to go more deeply.

7. *Intuitional/Compassionate Body-Divine Level: Medulla oblongata, the lower back of the head at the base of the skull.*

Opening this chakra stimulates divine understanding and lifts awareness to being one with God. The negative side of this chakra is that you could get caught almost exclusively in an awareness of mundane life. Massage the chakra. Where in your life do you most sense a divine plan and truly feel a oneness with God? You may feel a peaceful bliss awareness. Then ask the chakra where you block destiny; this will sometimes elicit an "oh-oh" response.

Will/Spirit Body

1. *Will/Spirit Body-Physical Level: Palms of hands and soles of feet.*

Energy from here helps a person relate with the outside world. These are some of the strongest locations for healing energy. Massage the hands and feet. Let the energy flow out of each of the chakras. Where does it seem most blocked? Walk around for a few moments (barefoot is best), feeling the energy connecting with the floor or earth. Be aware how the rest of your body reacts; usually there is a sense of coming alive. You may then wish to sit down and open the energy more in your hands. Hold your hands out four to eight inches from your body, then move them over your body and feel energy from the palms of your hands relaxing and healing your body. You may notice more energy if you hold the right hand over the left side of the body, then left hand over the right side of the body; this provides an extra polarity and may increase the energy.

2. Will/Spirit Body-Emotional Level: Backs of knees and insides of elbows.

Many people have emotional concerns—fear, a sense of inadequacy—about using the powerful will/spirit body. Enter a meditative state and massage behind your knees and inside your elbows. What frightens you or makes you uneasy? Visualize yourself doing well in these situations, and the energy flowing out in a beautiful, healthy way.

3. Will/Spirit Body-Mental Level: Armpits and where legs connect on the front side of the body.

Massage these chakras. Be careful not to massage any swollen lymph glands too hard (most people are too ticklish under their arms to massage that deep). Let the energy flow. Feel the strength in your body, a sense of power and spirit as it flows through your entire body when these areas are opened up. You may wish to walk around for a few moments, feeling these chakras open and flowing. Then enter a meditative state and visualize yourself using these places of power to help you in your daily life.

4. Will/Spirit Body-Intuitional/Compassionate Level: About an inch below the crotch.

See the seventh level of this body, of which this chakra is a companion.

5. Will/Spirit Body-Will/Spirit Level: Power sex chakra, two chakras below navel.

This is the most intense of the sex chakras and concerns not only sexuality, but sexual energy as it is turned into power. Many people block this chakra off without realizing it. Enter a meditative state and massage. Be as honest with yourself as you can. Do you like to control others? Do you feel you do so? If so, is it in a healthy or unhealthy manner? Do you like controlling others with your sexual energies? When have you let others control you with theirs? After finishing the meditation, feel the peaceful, beautiful and strong energies coming from the chakra and develop an awareness of how they affect the rest of your life.

6. Will/Spirit Body-Soul Level: Behind crown chakra at top of head.

A depression at the top of the back of the head may indicate that your pineal gland is working very well. Sometimes this chakra is open like a small dish. It aids in communication with higher dimensions and obtaining bliss states. Massage the chakra; let energy flow. Using deep peaceful breaths, get the feeling of floating in your body, then ask to be open to the bliss state. This may take some practice. Upon finishing the meditation, bring the energy back into your body and let your entire body feel a state of bliss. Stretch very well so that you connect your energies together (bliss may be nice but it is a difficult base to function from sometimes). Because of the power of this exercise, do not stay in it for more than a few minutes in the beginning.

7. Will/Spirit Body-Divine Level: Four fingers' width above the crown chakra.

This chakra, smaller than the crown chakra, is where human and spiritual energies combine. From a very comfortable position— lying down is best—be aware of the area above your head and the area below the crotch (the level four chakra of this body). Let the energies spiral outwards from these chakras. Experiment with the direction of the spiraling. When the energies have flowed for a few moments, enter a peaceful meditative state. Ask to be connected to the cosmos energy. Do not stay in this exercise for more than a few minutes in the beginning as it can be quite powerful. When your meditation is complete, stretch well.

Soul Body

1. Soul Body-Physical Level: Four chakras; on the instep of each foot and on the thumb side of the wrists.

These chakras concern the action of your I-AMness. They help bring consciousness to your hands and feet so you can be more aware of your actions. Here you can walk with a firmer step, taking action from your soul level. (There is a prayer I like for this level to bring you strength, awareness and direction: ask that the soul come in and work through your personality in your body.) Massage these chakras; ask which situations seem to block them and your I-AMness. Which situations facilitate opening?

2. Soul Body/Emotional Level: Above the knees on the insides of the legs and just above the elbows on the insides of the arms.

These chakras relate to your feelings about your I-AMness or soul level. When they are blocked you tend to pull your arms closer to your body and your knees will generally be weak. Massage these areas. Let the energy flow through them and ask the strength of your soul energy to refine and cleanse your emotions. Ask what makes you close these chakras and what helps you open them.

3. Soul Body-Mental Level: On the front where the legs join the body just on the inside of the curve, and on the front edges of your armpits.

These I-AMness chakras allow you to open up to the more transcendent part of life and things that normally go beyond everyday living. It brings energy for exploring and perceiving new ways of being. Massage the chakras. Ask them where you could be more exploratory in life and where you have done well.

4. Soul Body-Intuitional/Compassionate Level: At the front of the gonads—the ovaries or testicles.

The energy from these chakras helps you feel and understand your polarity identity (maleness or femaleness). Its purpose is important, as so much of life is based on interaction between polarities. As we open up to our polarities, we function better. Be in appreciation of your polarity identity. Let the energy of the ovaries or testicles flow. You may feel some sexual feelings but that's all right. People need to be as relaxed and accepting of sexuality as they are of feelings, thoughts and spiritual energies. Many people are embarrassed about discussing polarity identity. Our inability to accept and work with polarity energy holds us back in many areas. Where do you hold back yours? Do you feel that you are not male or female enough? Where are you doing well with these energies?

5. Soul Body-Will/Spirit Level: Lower ribs.

These are companion chakras to the xiphoid process, relating to your place in the world and particularly concerning your willpower to take the breath of life, own the right to be, express through breathing and accomplish what you wish in life. Open your lungs. Give them space and really breathe. Massage these chakras and get the feeling that your whole chest comes up from them, that you do have the right to breathe. Then ask the consciousness of these chakras when you block them and when you open them.

6. Soul Body-Soul Level: On the side of the neck as it curves into the body.

These chakras relate strongly to self-respect and are very powerful. Closing them off may bring tension or lock in an attitude of pride. Fear of really allowing your I-AMness to come out can cause you to pull in your head turtle-style, an action which affects these chakras. Let the chakras be open and ask yourself where you need to relax to facilitate your ability to come from your I-AMness. Ask in which situations you tend to block this flow or open it.

7. *Soul Body-Divine Level: Above the ears, on the sides of the head behind the temples.*

These chakras relate to feeling yourself as a unit of God's consciousness connected with the universe. Blocked or non-functioning, they can leave you feeling isolated, alone and fearful of life. Some forms of mental illness affect these chakras. Massage them; let the energy flow. Let yourself be lifted up and feel yourself one with God, a unit of God's energy and consciousness. You are an individuated unit of consciousness, an individuated part of oneness. Be aware of the energy and spread it all over your body; then ask which situations help you feel this energy and which situations block it.

Divine Body

1. *Divine Body-Physical Level: Twenty Locations; the ends of the fingers and toes.*

The energy from these chakras can be used to heal and as little antennas to know when something is in front of you. Massage your toes and fingers to promote energy flow through the chakras. Take deep peaceful breaths and feel yourself becoming more connected with the energy around you. In what ways do these flowing chakras increase your awareness?

2. *Divine Body-Emotional Level: In the center of the back of the head.*

A person in a prayer state channels more energy out of this chakra than out of the crown chakra. Bowing to others—an energy of respect—also opens this chakra; so bow your head and let energies flow out the devotional chakra. Are you comfortable doing this? Some people find that this chakra is excessively open and that they may be devoted to others or to a cause out of balance with the rest of life. Or they may find that it is closed, in which case bowing the head might be uncomfortable and they may wish to find out where their minds are closed. Do you project your faults onto others? Are you plagued by feelings of paranoia? Massage the chakra. Let a peaceful flow of energy go from it and let yourself be devoted to your destiny, to oneness with others, the cosmos and to your divine source. After a few moments of this meditation let the energy permeate your entire body and return your head to an upright position.

3. *Divine Body-Mental Level: Just inside the pelvic bones above where the legs join the body, down on the corners of the belly area.*

Expressing thankfulness is a necessary part of a healthy life. Closed divine body-mental level chakras may cause problems with your intestines. Massage these areas, let the chakras be open and let the energy flow. Ask where you need to be more thankful in life and where you need to open up more to abundance. You may wish to spend a few moments just being thankful for everything.

4. *Divine Body-Intuitional/Compassionate Level: Solar plexus.*

This chakra is one of the most important at the beginning of the Aquarian Age, a time when we have so much freedom of choice. Massage the solar plexus chakra. Breathe into it and ask to know what you are blocking. Then ask to know where in life you should take more control and action.

5. *Divine Body-Will/Spirit Level: At the base of the throat where the bones form the shape of a horseshoe.*

Sometimes people are asked to do more for others than they are comfortable doing. Or people may demonstrate an excessive need to serve. It is easy to feel martyred from this chakra. Lightly massage it. Let the energy flow out and, with your consciousness in that chakra, ask where in life you feel martyred or are excessive about service. Also ask where in life you hold back.

6. *Divine Body-Soul Level: On either side of the navel.*

These chakras are companions to the navel. They help unify the body's energies with both divine energies and other people. Massage the chakras; then massage the navel to achieve a balanced flow. Let energies flow out. Where in life are you involved in an excessive search for oneness with others and where do you block a oneness with others? As energy flows out of these chakras, meditate on your relationships with other people and cosmic levels.

7. *Divine Body-Divine Level: On top of the head-crown chakra.*

This is one of the best known chakras. It has great importance in our growth and connectedness with higher levels. Massage your crown chakra. Feel the top of your head. Is it tight? Open it up and let the energy flow out. As it flows, feel a oneness with others and with your divine source. Put yourself in a meditative attitude with this chakra and be aware of energy changes, insights or spiritual experiences. When this chakra is excessively open you may feel a great outpouring of energy; in this case it is best to bring the energy down around your body and all or some of it back, diffusing it throughout your entire body for strength. Excessive flow from the crown chakra may weaken a person. If yours is excessively open, ask yourself what circumstances in your life caused this condition. It may be a fear of being human, or it may come from times of excessive anger.

Sounds in Kundalini Movement

Sound is a very important part of life. It activates energy patterns, releases blocks and increases the life flow. It also plays an important part in the release of Kundalini and the opening of chakras. Continued vibrations at a particular frequency create movement in the energy they touch; as certain sounds can shatter a glass, certain vibrations will activate the flow of energy in areas related to the same frequency.

Mantras
The following are Sanskrit words or mantras (thought forms) which relate to the chakras. Repeat these particular sounds five to ten times while concentrating on the related chakra. Several minutes for each in the beginning is sufficient. Either sit in the lotus position or lie down. Take three complete breaths before beginning. (It is all right to spend a longer time on some chakras than on others.)

Root—*Lam*
Sexual—*Vam*
Navel—*Ram*
Heart—*Yam*
Throat—*Ham*
Fifth Eye—*Om*
Crown—*Aum*

As a variation for the crown chakra, open up to "all sounds," or the hum of the universe. If you wish to visualize the seed mantras, the Jain version of the Sanskrit is shown below.

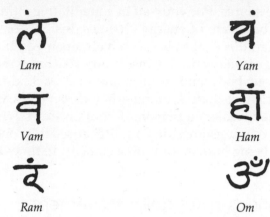

Lam

Yam

Vam

Ham

Ram

Om

Blissing out the Chakras

This is an excellent exercise for cleansing and vitalizing chakras and moving Kundalini. It is strong enough to cause a person to become sleepy or lose interest in completing the exercise; for that reason I recommend that only two chakras, the navel and crown, be used the first time. Add other chakras as your attention can handle it. At times the energy itself may pick the chakras it wishes to work on; let this happen. When finished, diffuse the energy throughout the body; never leave it concentrated on one area.

Omit the root chakra until all others are activated; doing the root before the others are open poses great difficulties, as there would be too many blocks and the main force would go down—not helpful to evolutionary progress.

Bring the energy up from the lower spine and out the opening of the chakra with which you have chosen to start. If the area feels stiff or blocked, massage it. Visualize a red flame burning out all the dross and negativity in the chakra, cleansing it for purer energy flow. There may be a variety of sensations, remembrances or thoughts; let them come, but do not hang onto or pay much attention to them. Let the red flame burn them and purify the area. The emotional or mental energies in some of the chakras will seem almost overpowering, especially for any of a sexual, emotional or lower mental nature. Do not let them take over. Visualize the red flame cleansing them.

After the burning, you may feel the energy begin to rotate in a clockwise manner (if looking at the body from the outside). Let this happen; the chakra is beginning its circular motion. After it has rotated for a few moments, let it extend out, still rotating, as far as possible. Even if the rotating sensation is not there, let the energy expand anyway and extend until it reaches the blissful state. Imagine your breath going through that chakra.

In the beginning, remain in this blissful state for no longer than five minutes. The energy is very high powered and your system is probably not used to it, no matter how good it feels. Remember, if you begin to feel tired, sleepy or bored, let the energy diffuse throughout the system and then quit for this time; do not do this exercise when you have trouble keeping interested or staying awake.

After finishing, let the energy disperse into the universe. Do not bring it back into the chakra; it is too powerful. Go on to the next chakra. It is best to start with the lower chakras and go up. At times it will seem natural to skip some that are normally done and go on to others. Eventually, do them all as described above. After doing the crown chakra, mix some of the energy with spiritual energy and let it shower over the body and come into the cells.

When all chakras have been cleansed and vitalized by the flame and the blissful state, do the root chakra. After that, be sure to bring the energy back into the spine and up and out the crown chakra, mixing it with spiritual energy and letting it shower over the body and through the cells. No matter how many chakras you do, always end with the crown chakra; you need the balance of the energy force. If you do the lower chakras last, the energy may get stuck there. Too heavy a concentration of energy in this area may cause physical, mental and emotional problems.

You may notice after a while that the three main focal points for energy—the navel, heart and fifth eye chakras—continue to clean themselves. Some may find that their third eye (between the eyebrows), activates instead. When the spontaneous cleansing occurs, do not interfere; open up to the energies. If possible, also take time for the blissing, a blessing and recharging force.

You may end this exercise by diffusing the energies in the body or taking them to the crown chakra and combining them with the divine energies, letting the combination shower over your system.

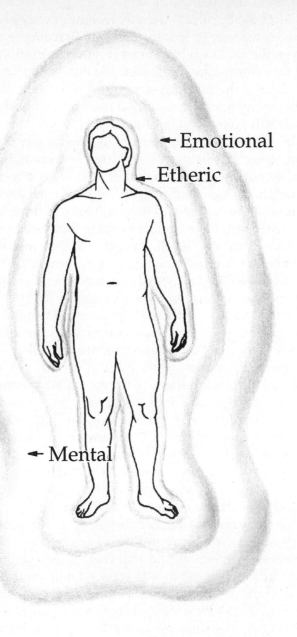

Etheric, Emotional, Mental Bodies.

Chapter 9

Measuring Chakra Flow
for Personality Reading

Chakra Measurement

In this chapter we will explore the effects of flowing or blocked chakra energies on personality and behavior using the seven main chakras and seven lesser-known chakras. There are many more chakras, and for a more in-depth reading they could be measured; but the general personality is expressed through these fourteen.

Chart 3 is a list of the fourteen chakras and their locations. Measurement is recommended for only the three lower bodies (physical, emotional and mental); they mainly determine personality, while the higher bodies are hard to measure because of their size, subtle nature, and the difficulty in locating them when they are not well developed.

The illustration opposite shows a pattern of even and flowing body energies. The etheric body expands beyond the physical, the emotional beyond the etheric, and the mental beyond the emotional; these bodies interpenetrate the physical body.

It may take a little practice to locate the outer limits of chakra flow. The following exercises are designed for that purpose.

1/ Rub your hands together to create static electricity and heighten your sensitivity.

2/ Hold your hands as far apart as you can with your palms still facing each other.

3/ Slowly bring your palms toward each other. You may feel your first "wall" of energy within a few inches, like the edge of an invisible balloon, or you may experience a sudden warmth or

Chart 3—Energy Testing At Chakra Areas							
Chakra/Area	7	6	5	4	SP	3	S
Etheric Body							
Emotional Body							
Mental Body							

Front

7 — crown
6 — brow—5th eye
5 — throat
4 — heart
SP — solar plexus
3 — navel
S — spleen
2 — sex
T — toes—end of big toe
     under toe nail
F — feet—center of bottom

Back

1 — root
W — will
EH — escape hatch
D — devotional

Name:_____

Date:_____

Chart 3—Energy Testing At Chakra Areas							
Chakra/Area	2	T	F	1	W	EH	D	Aver.
Etheric Body								
Emotional Body								
Mental Body								

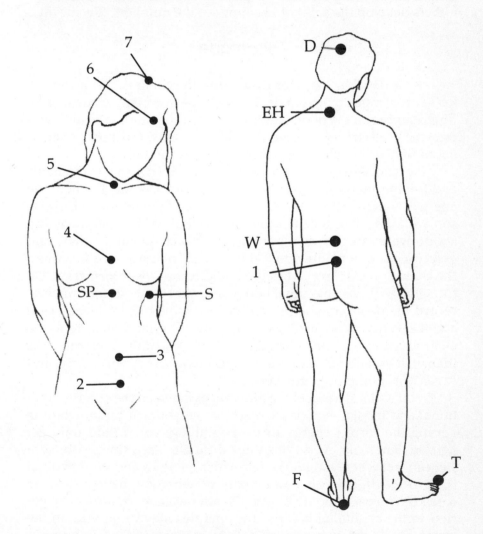

Energy Testing at Chakra Areas—Front and Back Views.

tingling in your palms. Strong energy may go up your arm. This is where the emotional body "wall" is found in most people.

It should be fairly easy to feel the energies this way as you are feeling them twice, once from each palm chakra. As you become aware of them you will notice their quality is different for each body level; a peaceful body may feel "smooth," while an irritated and agitated body may feel like and appear as fine silvery needles $1^1/_2$-2 inches long. Some people develop the ability to see the energy walls. Others develop the ability to hear or see the numbers psychically.

Technique

A yardstick is okay for measuring the chakras, but a carpenter's rule is much more handy. Have the person being measured lie down supine on the floor, hands at sides. Rub your hands until you feel static electricity. Locate the subject's physical body energy, about four inches above and around the entire body.

Next, locate the chakra to be measured. Stop for a few moments and feel the energies above it with your hand. Do not "bounce" the energy, as this disturbs the natural flow; and do not touch the person with the ruler, for the same reason. Pull your hand away, up about twenty inches, then put it above the chakra and slowly and gently come down until you feel the "wall" of the etheric body and the chakra on that level. Measure it and record the information. Do the same with the emotional body, only start at about forty inches; record the distance when you find it. For the mental level, begin about seventy inches away (you may need to stand on a stool or a chair; be careful, falling changes the energies, not to mention risks injury). If you do not find the chakras below the twenty, forty, and seventy inch marks, go further out.

You will learn to feel the differences between the etheric, emotional and mental energies. Do not hassle yourself too much over getting the correct energy in the beginning; you would only get nervous and make everything more difficult. Many times your subject can feel when you hit the particular energies and guide you in the process. If, later on, you wonder whether you have measured correctly, go back and do it over. Do not measure for too long a period in the beginning because the energies may drain you; in the event you do get "wiped out," a drink of water and a few minutes rest will generally refresh you enough to continue. Chakra flows

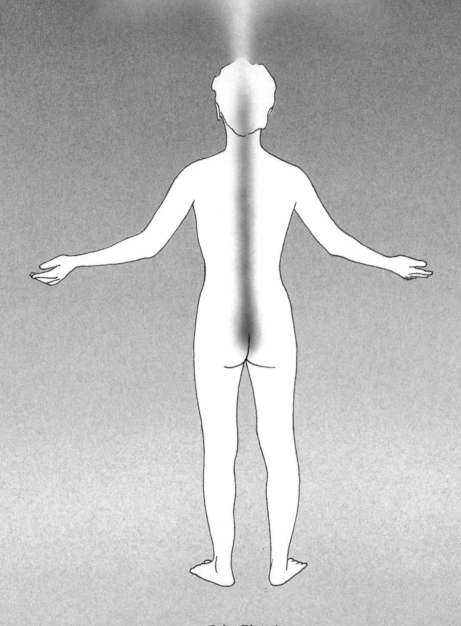

Color Plate 1
*The red-orange of the Kundalini rises up the spine and mixes with divine energy
(union of Shakti and Shakta). The colors turn golden, or sometimes silver.*

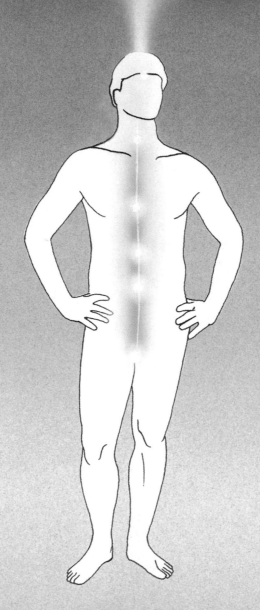

Color Plate 2
Imagine or feel the energy radiating from **Sushumna** ***and the*** **Chakras.**

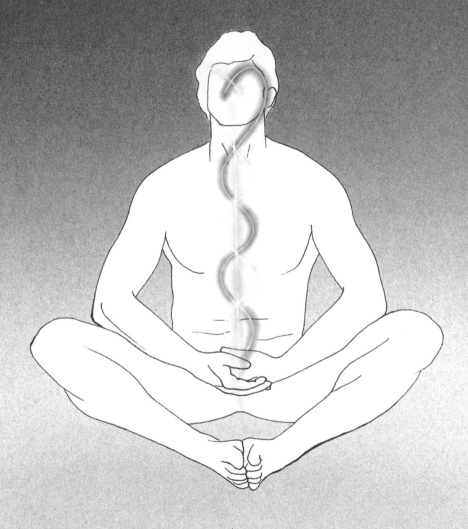

Color Plate 3
Pingala is silvery with a golden caste. It is masculine in nature. **Sushumna** is in
the spine, silvery with a bluish caste and has spiritual properties. **Ida** is silvery
with a reddish caste. It is feminine in nature. (See discussion, pp. 169–170.)

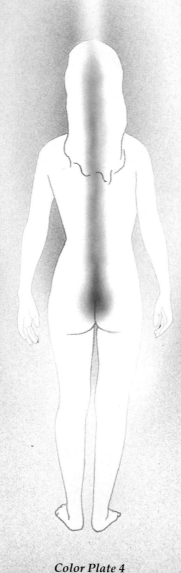

Color Plate 4
The red-orange Kundalini energy rises up through the body and out the crown chakra. It mixes above the head with the divine energy (radiant white or silver) and the mixture showers over the body in a luminous golden or silver sheen.

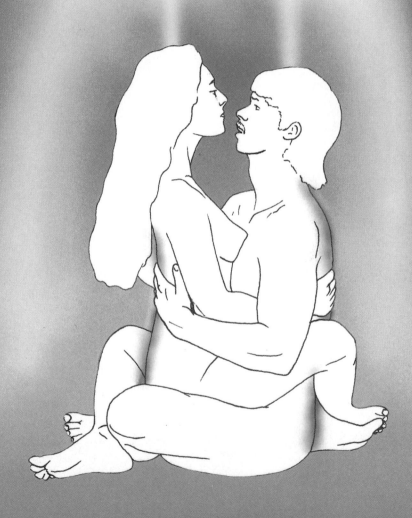

Color Plate 5
After preparation of the bodies, the Tantric Maithuna posture may be used
to raise Kundalini through sexual arousal.

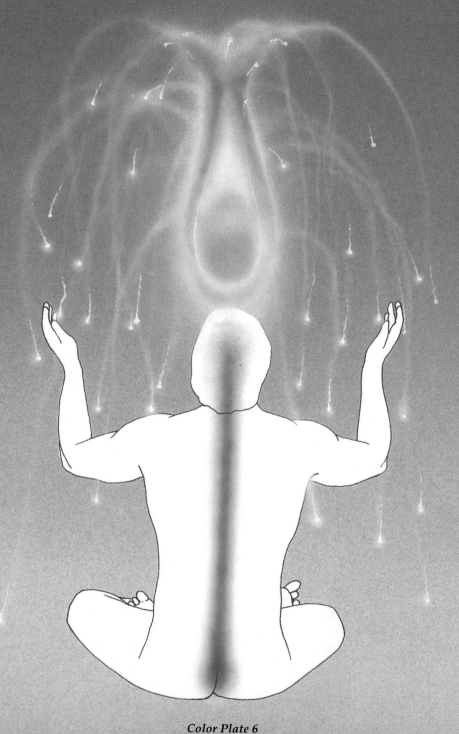

Color Plate 6
Imagine the Kundalini as a gentle, everflowing candle above your head. (You may wish to substitute an everblooming lotus blossom or rose.) When using the candle imagery you may wish to see or imagine the showering as sparks of light.

that you have trouble locating may be angling to the right or left or up or down; if so, make a note of it.

When you have finished with the front chakras, measure the back. After measuring, average the three flows (etheric, emotional and mental) and record the numbers on the chart. Now make a note of any significant variations within each level. A variance of one to two inches either way in the etheric is normal; three to four inches in the emotional, and five to six inches in the mental. Excessive variance means the energies are unbalanced and leads to confusion and mood swings. On the other hand, excessive consistency within any of the chakras indicates rigidity. In a truly balanced person, the higher chakras, such as the heart, fifth eye, or crown, are a little higher than the rest.

Be aware of the following while doing a personality reading:

1/ Energy flows vary somewhat from day to day. A general pattern may remain indefinitely if a person makes no effort to change.

2/ Extreme anger, hurt, love or any other emotion will show up in the energy flow. Comparing the measurements of extremely emotional states with those of fairly normal states will give you an idea what anger does to your system.

3/ Personality problems both cause and are caused by energy imbalance; it is difficult to know which comes first.

4/ Physical injuries may release energy or cause flow change.

5/ When a chakra is too open you may put your hand over it, push the energy back into the body, and mentally direct it to a chakra that is low.

6/ When a chakra is too low, massage it and the area around it; this will release any muscle tension, allowing you to send energy out that chakra mentally.

7/ Whenever you discover several walls or edges to a chakra, record the measurement farthest away from the body. Walls within walls indicate partial development of that body or chakra area.

Analyzing the Chakra Profile

Having measured and charted the energy flow of the physical, emotional and mental bodies through the chakra systems, we are ready to study the profile and find areas in which the subject may experience energy crisis. Personality problems are created by an

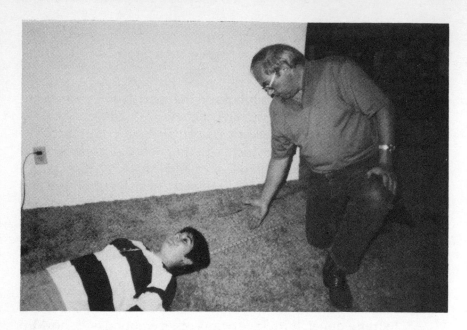

Photo 1: In this photo the crown chakra is being measured.

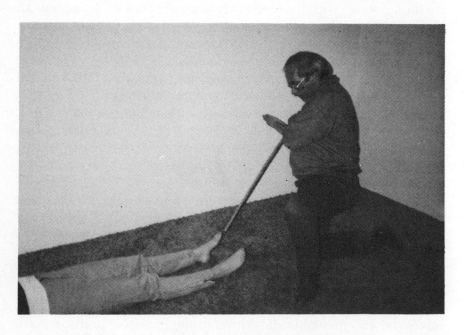

*Photo 2: In this photo the toe chakra energy is being measured.
Note the angling of the energy.*

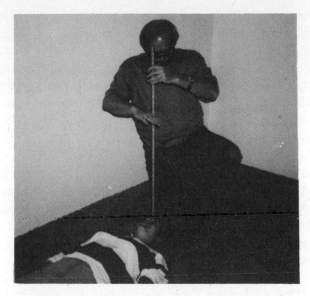

Photo 3: The fifth eye chakra flow is being measured.

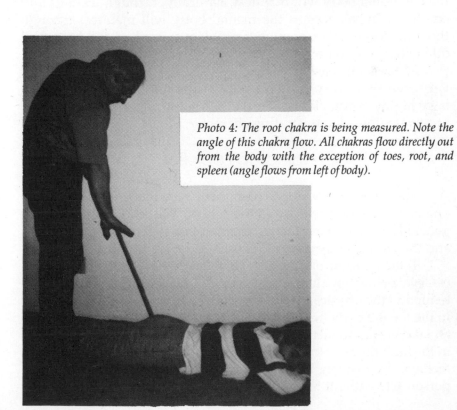

Photo 4: The root chakra is being measured. Note the angle of this chakra flow. All chakras flow directly out from the body with the exception of toes, root, and spleen (angle flows from left of body).

imbalance or disturbance of the energy flow within the physical, emotional and mental bodies. The chakra profile graphically shows in what areas these imbalances occur.

Any extremely above average chakra is probably too open and receives too much energy; or below average, is blocked and receives inadequate energy. (The symptoms of too much openness or blockage are described in Chapter 8.) Beyond the individual chakra measurements, it is important to look for particular patterns or relationships between chakras and bodies. There are many patterns of interaction that operate to create personality disturbances, but several common patterns may be noted. These general guidelines for analyzing a profile with reasonable accuracy may be noted:

1/ Look for the highs and lows in each body to determine where the energy is flowing too intensely and where it is blocked.what areas these imbalances occur.

2/ Imbalances in the chakra system of the physical body will manifest through both actions and physical illness. Imbalances in the emotional body will manifest, naturally, through feelings and emotions. Imbalances in the mental body will manifest through thought. When severe enough, a problem in one body will affect all other bodies in some way.

3/ General tension or rigidity usually indicates low energy, very even all the way around—not a healthy situation. It is better to have highly erratic flows; at least then some energy is getting out. Moderate flow, demonstrating character, is best.

Things to Look For

There needs to be good balance between the bodies. Be wary if one body is closed relative to the others. The etheric level should generally be above ten inches, the emotional above twenty inches and the mental body above fifty inches.

Take, for example, a mental level in the seventies and a physical level below ten; this indicates lack of follow through, lack of attention to the physical body, inactivity—in short, too much energy in the mental body means there is much more thought than action. Or take an emotional body in the forties or fifties with a mental body in the high fifties or low sixties; this indicates a preoccupation with feelings. Excessively high physical energies would suggest that a person acts without feeling or thinking.

When one chakra is very blocked, look to see where the excess is going. A blocked heart may go out the spleen in anger or out the sex chakra in excessive sexual energies. A low throat chakra suggests non-acceptance or resistance as well as an excessive flow out the heart chakra and a tendency to be overly loving. The energy from a blocked navel and spleen can go into the the sexual or root chakra.

A person excessively caught up in a particular problem generally gives extra energy to the associated chakra; that chakra may then become greatly opened, pulling the person's attention continually to it and only compounding the problem. It becomes a vicious circle. Try moving the energy away from a particular chakra to release the overload, or spread the energy from that chakra and your concern all over your body, diffusing the situation and bringing new awareness and new insight.

Excessively low crown chakra opens you to put-downs (from others or from yourself) and a fear of getting a big head. An excessively high crown, on the other hand, is usually all right, though it may release too much energy and blow open, resulting in general fatigue, a lack of energy for everyday pursuits, and a need to rebalance. In this case, try bringing some of the energy back and moving it throughout the body.

A high fifth eye chakra is all right unless it takes energy away from other chakras. It can indicate vivid dreams, clairvoyance—or headaches. Excessively low fifth eye indicates lack of vision.

Excessively high throat chakra suggests an overly accepting personality and a lack of reason. Excessively low throat indicates non-acceptance of life and an inability to speak up.

Excessively high heart chakra suggests that a person is too loving for his or her own good, may feel drained (burned out) or literally have heartaches. Excessively low heart suggests a downhearted or heartsick state, fatigue, depletion, and hard-heartedness; there may be great pain from earlier in life or from past lives.

Excessively high navel chakra produces an overly emotional state, leaving little energy to think or act. Excessively low navel indicates a blocked state or a fear of feeling.

Excessively high spleen chakra may result in uncontrollable anger and trouble thinking clearly. Excessively low spleen indicates a fear of expressing anger.

Excessively high will (if the heart is closed) naturally indicates a very willful state and a person who is difficult to get along with. Excessively low will usually indicates a pervasive sense of helplessness in which the energy spills into the emotional area. Will should be balanced with heart and navel.

Excessively high root chakra makes it difficult to sit still. A person could also be "sitting" on potential and repressing anger. Hemorrhoids may result. Excessively low root may produce a fear of mistakes. With head and root both closed, there may be a general fear of life leading to hiding (turtle complex).

Excessively high devotional (if higher than the crown) indicates devotion without direction, whether to a person or cause. Low devotional describes a person who is closed to others' ideas, inclines to project onto others, is preoccupied with the rights of self, and is suspicious of others.

Excessively open escape hatch chakra can leave a person spacey, especially when the head sticks out in front of the body too far. It closes off energy to the brain. In extreme cases, a person can feel paranoid. Excessively low escape hatch can mean overacceptance of the world.

Excessively high foot chakras indicate anger, the need to walk in order to clear emotions and mind, and a need to be heard and make a mark in the world (especially so when the heels hit hard walking). Excessively low foot chakras suggest pussyfootedness, fear of walking, walking on eggshells, fear of "standing on your own two feet," and a need to hang on. Toes excessively high produce a desire to release anger through kicking (to kick the way clear); when too low, the toes may curl from a pulling-in action, emblematic of a need for security, such as a bird hanging on to a branch.

With heart and emotional chakras excessively closed, a person tends to show love through sex. The sex chakra may also become excessively high due to overflow from other chakras; combined with higher emotional or mental levels, this results in more thought about sex than action. Excessively low sexual chakra suggests an inability to express sexually or to use this energy in other ways.

Nausea may result from either excessively high or excessively low flows from the solar plexus chakra. This extreme indicates problems in acting, feeling or thinking appropriately regarding one's destiny. Excessively open, there is a preoccupation with destiny and daily affairs; excessively low, there is a fear of assuming a place in the world or of not being open to manifestation.

Chart 4—Sample Chakra Measurements
(in inches)

	7	6	5	4	SP	3	S	2	T	F	1	W	EH	D	Ave.	
A	21	27	22	28	33	23	27	30	24	19	36	23	22	27	26	Etheric Body
	42	37	33	50	48	37	56	63	34	46	78	50	58	35	48	Emotional Body
	72	78	86	86	80	64	84	108	74	69	96	74	74	74	80	Mental Body
B	13	10	14	7	11	13	17	25	14	16	10	12	15	13	14	Etheric Body
	34	26	35	28	32	42	47	49	45	46	21	23	24	25	34	Emotional Body
	77	59	50	59	59	56	84	77	78	70	48	54	48	43	62	Mental Body
C	8	9	8	9	9	8	9	8	10	9	11	15	12	9	10	Etheric Body
	22	17	22	23	20	21	23	13	16	23	38	29	35	35	24	Emotional Body
	50	54	52	60	52	35	48	36	60	54	78	54	71	74	56	Mental Body
D	35	13	10	9	13	8	10	15	18	14	18	14	17	27	16	Etheric Body
	43	47	46	48	47	47	31	36	48	33	45	59	43	45	44	Emotional Body
	65	83	72	71	68	59	56	66	74	59	76	71	71	76	69	Mental Body
E	26	19	25	24	22	22	36	32	10	14	33	31	12	26	24	Etheric Body
	38	43	46	47	44	42	58	48	43	27	82	52	44	37	43	Emotional Body
	84	81	78	86	69	69	69	73	76	59	114	77	75	72	77	Mental Body
	CROWN	BROW	THROAT	HEART	SOLAR PLEXUS	NAVEL	POWER SEX /	SPLEEN	TOES	FOOT	ROOT	WILL	HEALTH ATTACHE	DEVOTIONAL	AVERAGE	

Sample Measurements

Chart #4 lists the chakra measurements for five people of diverse backgrounds. B and C have the lowest levels of the group; both are in structured and traditional professions. A, D and E have much more freedom for personal and spiritual growth; all three frequently do work with their spiritual energies.

A/ The highest chakra reading is on the spleen, mental level. This person was undergoing a lot of stress at the time. The crown is lower than the average (80), indicating imbalance and, in particular, lack of self-esteem. The overall scores are high, suggesting development; but a crown that is low relative to devotional indicates a need for more self-appreciation; the "lid" is on, inhibiting the crown's flow. The heart chakra higher on all three levels than the crown indicates A puts others' needs first.

B/ As noted, this person is in a traditional, overly-structured, stressful work environment, borne out by higher spleen readings on the etheric, emotional and mental levels. Devotional energy is lower than the average; dissatisfaction and separation only exacerbate stress and anger. B's crown chakra is above the average, indicating development.

C/ This person is in the most structured and rigid work environment of all. The readings on the escape hatch—a chakra so called because it serves as a general repository of excess energy during difficult times—are higher than average. There is consequently a strong escape desire, but the devotional energies on the emotional and mental level are higher yet, indicating that the person is trying to make things work. The devotional is much higher than the crown, meaning that the person does not spend enough time on personal pursuits. C's self-opinion could certainly stand improvement.

D/ Good mental development, but the crown and navel are too low. A low navel on the mental level indicates difficulty in processing emotions; and since it is also low on the etheric level there is trouble acting from the emotions. In terms of feeling emotions, however, this case shows much better balance. Devotional is higher than crown, indicating excessive devotion to other things and a need to take more personal time.

E/ There are high mental and emotional scores on the root chakra, suggesting that in spite of good development E is "sitting" on available potential, especially in regard to leadership. The emotional body measurement on the crown chakra is lower than average, while the etheric and mental are above average, indicating E does not have clear feelings about self, balance or enlightenment. When some measurements are high and others are low, there may be problems with using any of those energies. E's root is more than double the crown, truly indicating a state of sitting on feelings. The mental brow level is high for devotional, will, and foot, indicating clairvoyant abilities and the possibility of more vivid dreams.

Chapter 10

A Chakra Miscellany

Companion Chakras

The chakras on the front of the body have smaller companion chakras on either side which normally have a lower flow of energy. Their purpose is to help govern the amount of energy going through the main chakra and to determine how the energy is used; the ones on the right side of the body relate to attitudes or thoughts about how active the chakras should be, whereas the ones on the left relate to the feeling level of operation.

Introductory Exercise

Be aware of the line of main chakras and the line of companion chakras two to three inches on either side of it. Which feel open and which feel closed? You may wish to hold your hands a few inches over your body, move them down the companion chakras, first one side and then the other; which ones feel blocked? Companion chakras left of the belly affect the descending colon very heavily; those right of the belly affect the ascending colon. The chakras along the chest affect the lungs on either side. Companion chakras in the forehead area affect the left and right brain and psychic sight.

When you find a blocked companion chakra, let the energy flow out by lightly massaging it and the area around it. If massage is painful, send energy from the ends of your fingers or from your palms. Now be quiet; let your mind ramble, your feelings open. You may come to know what caused the block in the first place. If you like, fill the area with lavender, a manifestation of a healing energy frequency, which erases non-spiritual matters.

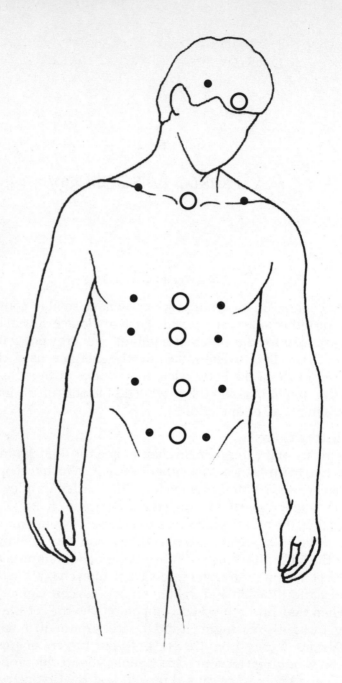

*Companion Chakras—note the smaller "companion" chakras
on both sides of the main or center chakras.*

Because this exercise may loosen powerful memories and images, healing yourself may be an overwhelming proposition. You may want to find a therapist or counsellor to assist you. It isn't necessary to do it all by yourself.

Three Sex Chakras

Sexual energy is a very important part of our Kundalini energy and can affect us in many ways, not just sexually. Though each of us relates to one sex chakra over the others, all three of the sex chakras need to be open and developed to ensure personal growth.

The three sex chakras lie between the navel and the pubic bone: the first 1-1$\frac{1}{2}$ inches (depending on body size) below the navel, the second the same distance down, and the lower at the top of the pubic bone. The energy from the upper chakra can be used in both creativity and sex; working well, it amplifies playfulness and joy, but working poorly it brings rigidity, humorlessness and lack of creativity. The flirtatiousness that may ensue may have a positive or negative result, depending on how it is used.

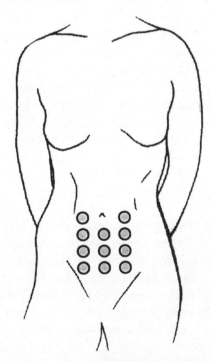

The companion chakras on both sides of navel and sex chakras.

The second sex chakra, next down, relates to power. Sexual union may empower people with strength and provide whole-body energy to establish a sense of inner stability, charisma and well-being. Though this energy has great healing potential, negated, it promotes a desire to control others with sex and results in people whom I call collectors—those fond of seeing how much sexual attention they can attract to themselves. Collectors have no interest in the positive side of the sexual energy. Rape is a manifestation of their imbalance.

The third sex chakra, just above the pubic bone, relates to transformational sex. Positive energy here transforms sexual energy to its higher octave, spiritual energy. People using energy from the third sex chakra may have visions and develop a new spiritual awareness. The negative side of this chakra manifests in a feeling that sex is evil and dirty.

Negative Chakras

Sexual energy is incredibly powerful, but excessive amounts in the companion chakras, without sufficient energy in the main chakras for balance, may result in a negative reversal (out the back of the body), leading to a savior complex, in which people feel they have answers to save the world. In extreme form, "saviors" feel destined to assert their agendas at any cost to individuals or society. Reversal may also be expressed as lust (insatiable desire) for sex, money, or power. Violence—against self or others—easily results from this condition, as a person is explosive and short-fused. When people aren't creative and don't change for the better, they become frustrated, feel there is no joy or control, and may react with criminal inclinations or other destructive avenues of self-expression. Some criminals are very creative, but their creativity has not developed positively.

It is my belief that in the future there will be chakra and Kundalini testing of children. Improper energy flow—too much to the companion chakras, not enough to the main chakras—may be caused either by a difficult childhood experience or by events from past lives. Physical and emotional abuse, suffering through traumas which undermine positive personal power and create feelings of helplessness and ineffectualness—these may split chakra energy flow and result in criminal behavior, poor learning energy and other problems. But counseling and redirection could be prescribed early.

The first step would be teaching the person to redirect the energy from these particular companion chakras inwards to the main chakras; the person then would learn to express through these chakras in more positive ways, to feel, for example, the energy of creative playfulness through the upper sex chakra or a positive self-affirming power through the power/sex chakra. A person would learn to feel the spiritual self, the transformation of the lower nature into more spiritual form. In severe cases a great deal of work would be needed, including professional help and supervision by a trained energy therapist. This would be necessary because of the incredible power the sex chakras can exert. Change would require vigilance. The person would be trained to balance these energies throughout the body so that excessive forces would not reside in particular areas of the body.

Seven Eyes[1]

Besides the two physical eyes to which we are accustomed, there are five additional spiritual eyes—all in our heads—that form a part of our expanded awareness or consciousness and open spontaneously in our travels on the evolutionary path. The third eye is

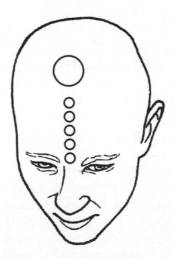

Location of the two physical eyes and five psychic eyes.
At the top, above the seven eyes, is the crown chakra.

---

1. This section is excerpted from *The Seven Eyes of Man in the Evolution of Consciousness*, by the same author.

located between the eyebrows; eyes four through seven are located on a line going straight up the forehead: the fourth just above the third, the fifth in the center of the forehead, the sixth just below the hairline and the seventh about one inch above the hairline. Each eye has its own particular function and all are needed in our complete development.

The two physical eyes have functions beyond ordinary seeing abilities. The first eye—the right—is primarily used to see the forms of objects; it aids in perception of detail. The second eye—the left—relates to our emotional self, more to color and texture than to form; it gives us a sense of the relationship between objects.

Our third eye gives us understanding of the form and workings of our physical world; it enlarges on what the first eye sees and brings depth or a third dimension. Open, it brings height into perspective, alleviating fear of heights or of flying. Our fourth eye is for understanding relationships and developing a belief in God; it enlarges on what the second eye sees. Our fifth eye aids in understanding universal truths and ideals; with it we receive "concepts" and it is excellent for past life viewing. Our sixth eye is necessary for true inner sight and for understanding the essence and purposes of our lives. Our seventh eye aids in understanding the totality and purpose of the universe; through it we receive divine understanding and see radiant light and angelic presences.

Few people have all seven eyes developed; few, in fact, have even the first two eyes fully developed. This is mainly due to ignorance of the possibilities in the various forms of sight, our laziness in comprehending or "seeing" what our eyes actually view, and insufficient regard for our spiritual heritage of expanded consciousness. All of these attitudes put veils over our eyes; but when we remove them, new worlds open up.

The Danger of Premature Opening

There are dangers in premature opening, the main one being lack of comprehension and fear of what isn't understood. People's eyes may "blow" open prematurely through drugs, physical injury (a head blow, for example), or through uneven development of the evolutionary process. Whatever the reason, when an eye opens without one's full understanding of its purpose, confusion and misunderstanding result; what should be a blessing may feel like a curse.

The Subconscious Eye

Also called "First Consciousness" Eye. The subconscious eye is located at the top of the nose, at the indentation below the bones that rise up to form the brow. It is an area of combined physical and emotional consciousness and as such relates to our basic or primitive living, gut level feelings, basic survival, and awareness. With this chakra open, it puts a person in touch with the subconscious (which is not supposed to be subconscious at all). Any emotional or physical difficulties which a person chooses not to deal with on a conscious level produce blocks, inhibiting growth and awareness.

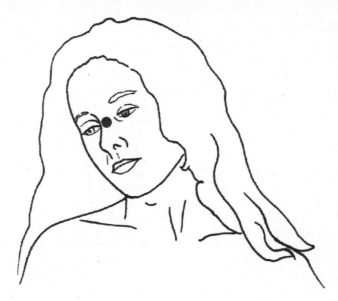

The subconscious eye is located on the nose between the eyes.

When the chakra is too open, a person suffers preoccupations with physical and emotional matters; too closed, and the person is out of touch with the life force.

An indication that this eye is beginning to open—that subconscious information is coming to awareness—is an urge to massage the area.

The Seven Hearts[2]

The seven heart chakras are all powered by the heart center. Each has a different kind of loving energy. They line up one on top of the other beginning at the xiphoid process and, for average sized people, are silver dollar size (if you are very small, the spacing will be closer; if you are very large, further apart).

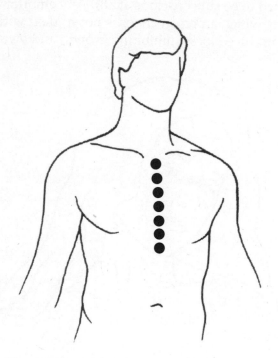

The seven heart chakras are "fueled" by kundalini
which is influenced by energy from the heart

---

2. Contributions to the text of this section and the Meditation are by Helen McMahan.

Heart Chakra #1

Location: on the xiphoid process, the bony appendage at the end of the breastbone.

Function: conscience energy; determining right and wrong.

Too open: guilt-ridden, defensive, rationalizing

Blocked: not aware of guilty feelings; impressionable.[3]

The very bottom heart chakra functions as your conscience, the little gyroscope of memory from all the early or sometimes late teachings which built up the *oughts, shoulds* and *musts.* Your parents were the very first contributors to this storehouse of thoughts, but many other people, including you, have added to it: teachers, friends, spouses, other relatives, even culture itself, have prevailed upon your heart with these strictures.

Heart Chakra #2

Location: just above the xiphoid process.

Function: maintaining a balance of released energy in terms of connectedness with others.

Too open: over-attachment to a person or ideal, leaving little understanding or energy to balance the heart forces.

Blocked: rejects attachment; closed heart.

The second heart relates to attachment: to people, things, and ideas. There is often a cloying, dangerous, and heavy energy here, especially in a relationship. Remember that you cannot lovingly own, possess, manipulate or control another human being. The positive side to attachment is a deep caring, an acceptance of responsibility, a willingness to put yourself out for someone.

Heart Chakra #3

Location: on the breastbone between the breasts.

Function: will to live well.

Too open: impulsive, heedless.

Blocked: fear of life; weak will.[4]

The third heart chakra is the main one we work with in our basic Kundalini—the chakra of love and the will to live. Your heart here is your life, your driving force to embrace your life, enjoy it, learn from it, use it to grow personally, to discover your divine origins and return into that ocean of love that is the energy of God.

---

3. See also Emotional Body-Intuitional/Compassionate Level, p. 95.
4. See also Physical Body-Will/Spirit Level, p. 94.

Heart Chakra #4

Location: above heart chakra #3.

Function: forgiveness, letting light shine.

Too open: overly forgiving; accepting even when it means injury or damage.

Blocked: seeks vengeance; forces greatness or accomplishment on others.

The fourth heart chakra concerns vengeance and forgiveness. Forgiveness is an incredible blessing, both for the one who gives and the one who receives. Vengeance is the flip side; tightness and an inability to flow or let go result in a fierce and powerful desire to get even, to hold back, to block the true feeling of love.

Heart Chakra #5

Location: midpoint between the horseshoe in the neck and heart chakra #3.

Function: will to live; equilibrium, compassion.

Too Open: people pleasing.

Blocked: hard-hearted.[5]

The fifth heart chakra is your compassionate heart. Flowing, it will cause people to open to you like flowers; they may even start telling you all their troubles, attaching themselves to you like emotional vacuum cleaners. It can suck you dry. If you ever find yourself in this situation, imagine unplugging that energy from your heart and re-plugging it back into their own navel or a heart chakra.

Heart Chakra #6

Location: just below the horseshoe shaped bone in the front of the neck.

Function: to open to higher spiritual levels; to put heart energy into spiritual growth.

Too open: a tendency to see things only in higher levels or spiritual ways and ignore the more human lot in life.

Blocked: fearful; rejects higher spiritual levels.

The sixth heart chakra opens you to higher spiritual growth, spiritual melting, the outpouring of spiritual love you feel for your God. True love that we feel for others is very similar to this feeling. A person whose flow is too open, however, can be a pain, indulging in spiritual platitudes and inattentive to others' reality. Someone whose flow is blocked stubbornly sees only the human side of life.

---

5. See also Emotional Body-Divine Level, p. 98.

Heart Chakra #7

Location: where the bones in the bottom of the neck form a horseshoe shape.

Function: service in the world.

Too open: a person pushes to serve even when it's neither needed nor welcome.

Blocked: self serving.

The seventh heart is the service chakra. To give service is a high goal. When the energy of the seventh heart is blocked or twisted, it becomes a martyr's, a begrudging, mean-spirited, unacceptable giving which does damage to all concerned, much like a person "helping" the old woman across the street. Twisted energy can produce a martyr, someone who gives service to others but complains about it. Someone whose flow is blocked may be oblivious to opportunities to help others. But when flowing properly, this service chakra becomes a supreme purpose of this lifetime.

A Meditative Exercise on the Seven Hearts

Carefully massage the lowest heart chakra. If it is sore, you could injure it, so be very gentle. Relax; let your breath float deeply and gently into your body, watching it from that still, quiet space deep within you. Free your mind. Without fear or worry, open your memory. Look at your energy.

Ask what *shoulds*, *oughts*, and *must dos* are buried within this conscience heart chakra. Which ones are no longer valid and need to be laid to rest? As each stricture surfaces to your conscious mind, recognize your feelings about it, how each helps or hinders your ability to relax, relate, enjoy yourself and your life. What can you release? What should you enforce even more?

Move your awareness up to the chakra of attachment and non-attachment, next in line. Massage the area. Feel the flow of energy; notice its quality and recognize the feelings, ideas, essences of what this heart elicits within you. Ask yourself what you need, crave, love, or possess. Perhaps they are material things—house, car, clothing, some old trinket carefully cherished. What do these attachments mean to you? Or perhaps the attachments are to people, ideas, ways of relating to the world, ways of perceiving the ideal. What do these attachments do to your life? Do they free or restrict you? Comfort or cause you anxiety? Where do you really want to attach and what do you want to let go of? Can you watch yourself expand well beyond these cherished attachments?—loving responsibly yet letting go at the same time!

Open the will-to-live chakra—the major heart chakra in the middle of your chest between your nipples. Feel the powerful flow of energy from this strong, piercing chakra of love, the joyousness, openness, curiosity, and excitement for the next adventure. Let the energy pour out to embrace the next teaching or lesson; coax yourself; sift the lessons of your life for their kernels of truth, patiently allowing modification of existing love, knowledge and understanding. Let yourself simply experience who you are.

Now open the heart chakra of vengeance and forgiveness (directly above the will to live); experience the energy, notice the changes, and relax, letting the chakra flow. Are there old and deeply buried grudges here? What burdens can you let go of? What forgiveness can be released from this chakra? Breath deeply, peacefully. See in your mind's eye the face of the person with whom you have had the most difficulty in this life (whether now living or dead). Hear his or her voice. What is the most irritating thing that person does? Did you love this person? Does that love continue? Go back in your memory and determine the basic cause of the first difficulty you had with this person. Have you ever wanted to strike that person?—even kill? Any particularly irritating physical characteristics about this person? You may have felt there was another kind of relationship between you (for example, mother or father), one which does not exist in this life. Now forgive yourself for anything you might have ever said or done to this person. Take thirty seconds; say over and over again "I forgive myself" for whatever you may have done to this person. Now ask for God's forgiveness for any attitude you might have had, or anything you've ever said or done to this person. One half minute—God's forgiveness—ask it!

Silently now in your mind forgive this person for anything he or she may have done to you—specific acts, specific words. Forgive them now. One half minute, just forgive. And now for one half minute, pray for this person; send love to this person, bless this person—even if it scrapes your nerves raw—pray for this person.

Now relax. Smile. And flow from that sweet place of forgiveness within.

The next chakra up is the compassionate heart chakra. Massage it, gently focus the awareness, open the chakra, let your compassion flow out. Just feel the compassion; let it out indiscriminately for everyone who brushes against your being, your life. Compassion for your friends, for your family, for your intimates, and then for yourself. Flow over with the sweetness of compassion, letting yourself taste the humor of your compassion. Focus the power of this energy now totally toward yourself; let it wash over your quirks, foibles, pet peeves, secret habits; let yourself smile at this groping, curious, shining miraculous being that is you. Move on up now to the next heart chakra, that of opening up to higher spiritual energies, just below the horseshoe of your throat. Let a prayer form within this flow of energy—what does this opening to your divine origins feel like? Let your prayer form into a wish for a new start on life, a higher dedication of your spirit to a brighter calling. Check your wish for shreds of oughts and ought nots, for attachments that bind, for willfulness and ego, for hidden grudges, and pet likes. Now polish your wish, shine up this prayer, and let it go up into the divine.

Last, move your awareness into the hollow of the throat, into that horseshoe, the chakra of service. Let yourself concentrate on totally opening, expanding, breathing past the slightly choking, blocking, closing feeling that happens so easily in this delicate area. Ask what kinds of service are opening up in your life right now? Where are you making the effort to give to life? What does your service energy feel like? Notice it, experience it, sense it with all your being. Now ask what new areas of service are starting to open within you. Ask to experience the very highest that is in you to give. "I will to will Thy will." Form that intent, send it up, rededicate yourself to the seeds of service beginning to sprout within you—"I will to will Thy will."

Ring Around the Chakra Sets

Ring Around The Crown

"Ring around the crown" chakras may not be a very elegant description, but that is just exactly what they are. Six of them, found around the crown chakra (center of the top of the head), are listed below:

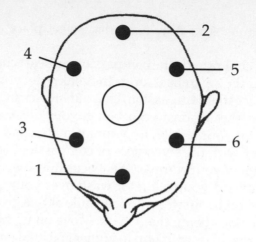

Ring Around the Crown Chakras—
The center is the crown, the others form the ring.

1/ This is the same as the seventh eye. (You may refer to seven eyes for further description, page 129.)

2/ Located in the back of the top of the head (some people may feel a depression there which can indicate a more developed pineal gland). This chakra is the same as the sixth level of the will/spirit body. You may refer to page 68 for further description.

3, 4, 5, 6/ These chakras are on the sides of this ring, two on the right side and two on the left. They relate to higher states of consciousness and receive information from higher levels, just like antennae.

You should work with the first or second chakras separately. Treat chakras three through six as an entire unit. Massaging the chakras (running you fingers around your head), you may notice changes in energy where the chakras are located. Measuring equal distances from one to three, three to four, four to two, two to five and five to six helps you in spacing them. Having massaged them, let the energy flow, making sure that it is also flowing from your crown chakra so you maintain a better balance. Imagine you are floating and be open to any information or ideas. Do not judge these thoughts for now; just write them down. Check them out later for meaning and how they illuminate your life.

Ring Around the Heels

"As above, so below." That's how it is—the "ring around the crown chakras" matches the "ring around the heels chakras." There is even a chakra in the center of the heels which corresponds to the crown.

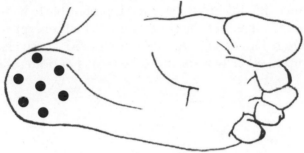

Ring Around the Heels—The center relates to the crown chakra.
The others relate to the chakras encircling the crown chakra.

These chakras do not receive a lot of attention but they are very important. Their purpose is to ground your spiritual experience and awareness and make it usable. With both the crown and heel chakras open, your head is in the heavens and your feet on the ground. We should remember that earth is part of the heavens; the "ring around the heel chakras" relate to cosmic power and energy as it manifests in the earthly realm.

Exercise
Find an open area where you can walk around. Massage all of the ring around the heel and head chakras. Walk around feeling the energy going through both the heels and the head. Be aware of the connectedness and the power in this combination. After a few minutes you may wish to sit or lie down (either way, keep your back straight). Enter a meditative state and be open to any images or thoughts that come to you.

For beginners, these chakra sets are not that important; but a person growing in the amount of spiritual force available needs to have these chakras open and balanced in order to make maximum use of it. These chakras also help maintain the physical body at a degree of strength where it can handle the power of the higher energies.

Shoulder Blade Chakras

These chakras are located just inside the center of the shoulder blades. When open, they energize your system and open you to higher learning. When closed, you may think of massaging them, but of course it is difficult to massage that area yourself. You may rub up against the side of a door, but it is preferable to have someone else do the massage. Let them be open. Which energies have you been blocking? How could you be more open? These chakras may open you up to other worlds and other ways of doing things.

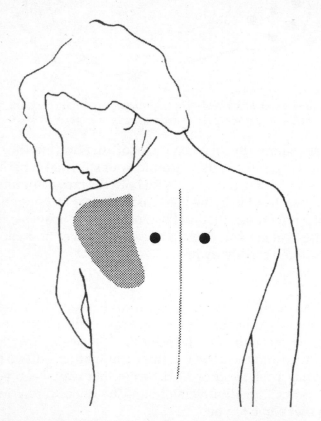

These shoulder blade chakras are just inside the shoulder blades.

Unity and Destruction Chakras

These are companions to the navel chakras (see page 125) and are similar except that the left one deals more with emotions and the right one more with thoughts. When the energy from these chakras is flowing well and positively out the front of the body, you have a sense of unity among the different bodies as well as between the entire body system and divine energy.

Energy from blocked unity and destruction chakras goes out the back and can be very destructive indeed. A person with such blocks is generally unaware of their destructive part not only in his or her life but in the lives of others. If you think you are destructive or cause problems, you may wish to check these areas and bring the energy frontwards to turn it into unity. It does not matter whether you are aware of the destruction caused from these chakras. It is your energy and you can still cause karma with it. Excessive energy can be brought to the navel for a peaceful feeling across the entire area.

Knee and Elbow Chakras

Knees

Find the indentations just to the outside and inside of your kneecap. These chakras concern showing reverence, bowing the knee either to the divine or to someone royal or a spiritual entity ("genuflection" literally means "knee bending"). The state of flexibility in your knees affects your entire body, and for that reason as well these chakras are important.

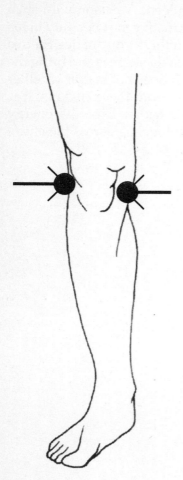 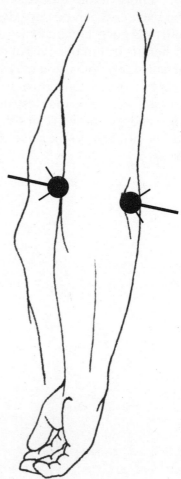

The chakras on either side of the knees relate to flexibility and devotion.

The chakras on either side of the elbows are similar in purpose to the knee chakras.

Elbows

These chakras, on either side of the elbows, are similar in purpose to the knee chakras. There are very open when a person puts his or her hands together in prayer. In fact, the prayer state—bent knees, palms together (bent elbows), and lowered head—opens the devotional chakra and allows great openness to higher, more spiritual realms. The body joins in the prayer with its energy, enhancing the spiritual connection. Blocked elbow chakras lead to great self-centeredness.

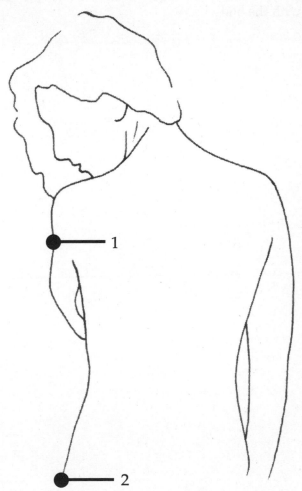

The body confidence chakras are located on both sides of the body, for a total of four. They are very important for a sense of well-being.

Body Confidence Chakras

These four chakras, two on the upper arms and two on the upper thighs, when balanced and open, give a sense of physical well-being, support through the body, and body confidence. Massage these areas. Let the energy flow in a balanced way. Take a few moments. Feel good about yourself and being in your body. With the body confidence chakras too open, a person is overly preoccupied with the body and its well-being; too closed, and a person will be out of touch with the body.

Chapter 11

Chakras and Relationships

Introduction

Because our chakras continually receive and send out energy, we are continually being affected by and affecting others, sometimes in positive ways, sometimes not. No wonder some people want to be hermits.

If your energies are strong, you will have an immediate impact upon anyone who comes into your presence. Specifically what kind of impact will depend on the condition of the other person's energy system. Someone who has weak energies or is not feeling well may be intimidated, overwhelmed or wiped out in your presence; that person also could be energized by you. If the other person also has strong energies, there is likely to be better balance and a better rapport—a feeling of being equal.

We experience energy primarily through our most open chakras. If your sexual chakra is the most open, then regardless of what you receive from others, you will experience it on the sexual level. Not only that, but the other person's energy will primarily go out the sexual level. If your heart chakra is the most open, you tend to experience life as love.

Energy received by overly open spleen or navel chakras will cause emotional reactions. Some people receive most energy through their third or fifth eye; they deal with the world primarily on a mental level. The unexpected reactions of others are due to this chakra "snagging" process; more on this later. The reverse also true; you receive strong energies from others through your strongest chakra. When you become aware of a strong reaction to another person but do not understand that reaction, seek to know the area or chakra of your body where you feel this energy most strongly. If you think your energy response is inappropriate, consciously move the energy to a different chakra area (such as the heart or brow).

When you become aware that your energies are too intense for comfort, stretch your body and breathe deeply. This breaks up the stress pattern and increases energy flow. Another way to achieve balance is to send energy out your feet and the top of your head. Dancing equalizes energy throughout the body and is therefore a good release when you feel pent up or blocked; it can also be used as a preparation for meditation or intense mental work.

Energy Ties

People who have strong mutual feelings establish energy ties which bind them even when they are not physically together. The bind may be at the heart, brow, navel, or sexual chakras, or combinations of the chakras. Those who are very sensitive to these energies can feel them, and the clairvoyant can see them. Two people who care deeply for one another but ignore each other when in the company of others might suppose they are hiding their connection; still, the bond between them can be felt or psychically seen.

When one person of a married couple starts sending energy to a third person, his or her mate may notice something is missing, suspect an affair is brewing, or feel a sense of loss and not know why. The reason is the diminished flow in the couple's energy connection.

In marriage or close friendships a strong tie can be very beneficial and comforting. When there are connections at all chakra levels, the partners have a feeling of blending and really fitting together. Relationships with an easy flow and strong contacts have a stronger chance of lasting. But intensity can be overwhelming. Too strong a tie may represent a loss of individuality. Sometimes one person takes on characteristics of the other. This is one reason we should be careful with whom we have our deepest contact.

Sometimes a parent will feel closer to or love one child more than another. This may stem from a strong past life connection, or may be due to chakra energy rapport in this life. Even when the parent tries to treat all the children alike, the other siblings usually sense who receives the most energy attention. They may insist the parent likes the other child better when actually there is only a stronger connection. Such connections can and do change during lifetimes. Negative feelings between people often manifest in a hatred connection between their spleen or navel chakras.

Exercise. Close your eyes. With whom do you have psychic ties? Are they negative or positive? Where do you feel them in your chakras? What are your ties with the other person's chakras? Do these ties drain or reinforce you?

Charisma and High Energy People

Charismatic people have strong energy fields which they can use in positive or negative ways. Have you ever listened to a speaker whom you thoroughly enjoyed only to wonder later how you could have agreed with the person's ideas? You were under the speaker's "spell," feeling a charismatic energy while in his or her presence. Great speakers can send the essence of their message through their energy and really touch their audiences, sometimes inspiring them. Great actresses and actors do the same thing. So do con artists. A charismatic person has the ability to send energies from different chakras which can snag the chakras of others.

Sometimes you will find that other people literally blow your mind with their forceful energies. You may be at a loss to answer the person, think clearly or verbalize your thoughts. You feel defenseless. This type of person usually sends very strong energies from the third eye (between the eyebrows) or the fifth eye (in the center of the forehead). If you find this happening to you, send energy out either your third or fifth eye, whichever seems appropriate, and let it meet the other person's half way; you will keep your thought patterns from getting messed up. If you find it difficult to follow or comprehend a speaker, send energy gently out your fifth eye.

Some charismatic people are so filled with love and peace that they seem single-handedly to change the vibrations everywhere they go. Just being in their presence others can experience the elevating effect of their energies.

Chakra Snagging

Another's strong energy flow from a particular chakra may snag you in that same chakra. Being with someone who is very irritable and upset may snag you; you become irritable and upset yourself. You may wish to send peace from your navel chakra to counteract the other person's energies. You may also find that concentrating on a higher chakra will help to balance things.

We all have to be careful of being snagged, careful too of what we send to others. One person in a crabby mood can set off everyone else, whether at home or work. Co-workers often leave a negative situation only to go elsewhere and complain about it, unaware they got snagged with the negativity and are spreading it. A wonderful gift you can give to other people is to let them have their space and not get caught in their moods or acting as if you caused them; likewise, you can feel your own moods without feeling compelled to snag others into it.

Children, especially, can snag their parents with their negative thoughts and emotions. Adults may give children their own way or totally shut them out as ways of getting them to stop snagging the chakras. Living together creates a situation where all people in a group tend to block or open the same chakras. Children pick up many of their parents' attitudes and feelings, even on a subliminal level, getting clues that certain chakras should be closed or open at certain times; without anyone's realizing it, the child takes on the parents' ways of relating to the world.

Every thought and feeling you have about another person becomes an energy form which goes to that person. It affects the person on some level. Do remember that anything you send out eventually returns to you. You get what you give.

If you feel inundated with thoughts and feelings from others, imagine yourself surrounded with a psychic ultraviolet light. If the feelings or thoughts get stronger, they are yours; if they fade away, they are someone else's. You may even be aware of the person sending them or see his or her face. The person probably does not mean any harm. There are many careless thoughts and feelings which pollute our air.

Do Unto Others

When you want someone to have certain energies, such as confidence or peace, feel that in your energies and usually it will reflect in the other person. Sometimes you may be angry over another's lack of calm or peace, but this only makes matters worse.

Clarity

Feeling what you are thinking or saying helps you be aware of what you really mean. It also helps convey the essence of your message and you will be more easily understood.

Sappers

People with low levels of energy may unconsciously drain or sap energy from others. Such people have not learned to absorb energy from the surrounding air, instead pulling it predigested from another person; or they are so emotionally disturbed or physically weak as not to be able to pull energy in for themselves. "Predigested" means that the energy has already been brought in by another person and transformed to a usable frequency; it is an easy way out.

People who for no apparent reason make you feel drained or irritable are sapping your energy. Energy pulled from you leaves you weakened. You may feel your aura shutting down. When this happens, your energy comes back toward you and your body tightens. You may look for excuses to get away from the sappers. When you have gotten away and your energy truly becomes yours again, you may wonder why you acted as you did. Were you uncaring or too hasty? Should you have stayed? Guilt feelings may ensue, which an awareness of this sapping dynamic may help you understand.

Feeling drained, you may wish to become aware of the chakra or chakras from which energy is being pulled. You can then make the choice either to close the chakra or send energy to the other person. Sharing energy is a gift, and what you give strengthens you. But when the person to whom you send energy does not relax and come into strength, you may need to stop sending energy. Sometimes people become dependent on others' energies. When you choose not to send energy, seek protection by filling and surrounding yourself with a white light, consciously willing your own aura to be stronger and creating a force-field against draining influences. Another procedure is that of imagining a glass wall between you and the sapper.

Those Who Stir It Up

A person with highly charged or unbalanced chakras may seek stimulating conditions, such as arguments, which aid the release of these excess energies. Some people are happier when they have caused a commotion. Their needling and fight-starting may stimulate their own energy and release blocks, but neither does much for the other person. Gossip, heavily judgmental, is another form of stir-it-up release. In the company of someone who is trying to stir it up, try to remain peaceful and not get snagged. You may need to change the subject or ask the person not to talk meanly of others in your presence.

Sex

Preoccupation with sexual thoughts or feelings may stem from excessively opened sexual chakras. Whether or not a person in this situation is aware of it, others pick up the sexual energies, perhaps even to the point of supposing interest in a sexual encounter. This can be confusing. Make sure in this situation that your own sexual chakras are balanced or your higher chakras are open; you will be less inclined to take things personally.

Sometimes people with very high spiritual energies and blocked sexual energies will attract people with blocked spiritual energies and high sexual energies. It is an attraction of opposites; but we are also dealing with higher and lower octaves of the same energy and it may be that one person's very spiritual energies attract sexual responses from another. Seek protection by filling and surrounding yourself with a radiant light and feeling balance all over your body. Relationships and sex are best when all chakras are balanced, open and flowing well.

Blocking

We spend a great portion of our lives in relationships, surrounded by the energy others are sending out. It is important both how we receive others' energies and how our own energies are received by others. In the company of someone whose chakras are blocked, you may feel shut out, as if that person wants nothing to do with you. This may not be the case at all. The person may very much want interaction but is so used to having blocked chakras that to open them in your company is a frightening proposition; relationships in this situation can be scary and tense.

When you want to be more open, feel your chakras as relaxed, open, and receptive to others' energies. There are some very positive benefits to openness: a sense of connection, strength, cuddliness, or of not being alone in the world. When you want others to be more receptive of you, let your energies out in a peaceful way. Do not force them or the person receiving them may feel bombarded.

Better Understanding Your Chakras: An Exercise

Close your eyes. Imagine that a significant person in your life is standing in front of you or near you. Be aware how your body reacts to this presence. Which chakras open or close? You will feel relaxed where they are open and tight where they are closed. More aware of the movement of your own energies, you will be able to have more control and enjoyment in life. Remember that energy patterns change according to the situation and the people you are with.

Chapter 12

Chakras and Healing

Introduction

Energy going in or out of the chakras affects the muscles, the nervous system and the glands. In short, it affects the entire system, and so a blocked chakra can create problems in all surrounding areas. With open and flowing chakras, a person will feel vibrant and radiant, ready to love life fully. But with partially or completely blocked chakras, a person does not have full access to his or her energy, which leads to confusion, depression, an off-centered feeling, or just general miasma. Energies can become blocked by tightening muscles, poor posture, or holding back energy in chakras.

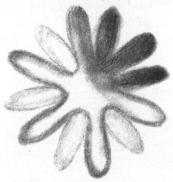

The darkness in part of the chakra may indicate negativity,
blocked energy or undeveloped petals.

151

Vibrant colors in a chakra indicate harmony and development. Dull or grayed and dark areas across part of the chakras indicate problems, whether non-development, negativity, fear of relating to the world, or physical, emotional or mental blocks. You may notice that some chakras are much more active than ones which surround them; people may over-emphasize a particular chakra and feed it by pulling energy from surrounding chakras. This leads to illness. On the other hand, blocking one chakra creates congestion in the entire area; blocking the sexual chakras, for example, out of fear of the sexual energy, may block the entire lower belly area, slowing all its functions.

People with low self-images tend to pull the energy in, in particular negative energy, since low self-image is negative. You may even take on others' maladies.

Too much unassimilated (hence, unusable) energy may bring a strong sense of inertia, lifelessness, or depression or a clogged, no-energy-to-cope feeling. Restlessness, irritability, and illness or ineffectiveness make up the basic pattern of this condition. Creative projects, physical exercise, and meditation help to assimilate and use blocked energy.

Chakra Blow-Out

Chakras may "blow open" in times of stress, up to a foot wide, too much for good energy use. Blow-outs occur with unmanageable energy and commonly affect the heart, solar plexus, and navel. Drugs may also blow the chakras open, most often the head chakras. The result of blow-out is ineffectiveness from the affected chakra and tremendous energy release that depletes the rest of the body.

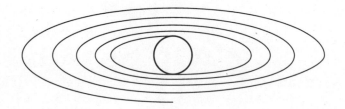

The circle in the center indicates where the chakra energy should be located.
The lines around it indicate the excessive opening which can come from fear,
excitement or other excessive feelings.

Try thinking the chakra back into a better position; if that does not help you may need professional assistance. You could also take your hand and gently go over the chakra three to four inches above the body, aiming excess energy back into the body. Move your hand clockwise or counterclockwise, whichever feels better.

Pain

Pain in a particular chakra indicates that the chakra is trying to open. Try very lightly massaging the area to help its release. If the pain continues, stop. Put your consciousness into that chakra, allowing thoughts and feelings to come to your awareness and opening you to discover what has been blocked. When awareness comes, pain or the block will generally disappear; but if it persists, it would be a good idea to get medical help.

Illness and Visiting the Sick

During illness it can be very helpful to receive energy from a visitor, especially when it is peaceful. Both the ill person and the sender are energized in the process. It is a beautiful partnership. An unthinking, unaware visitor, however, sometimes actually drains energy from the sick, worsening their condition.

A depressed person may benefit from receiving another's uplifting energy, but could also be hindered from going into and working on the depressing energies. A general awareness of energies and their flows helps you understand how to use your own energies more effectively with others.

When visiting the sick it is best to be as healed and whole in your own body as possible. The flow between you and the indisposed must be natural. Always allow energy to flow as it will; pushing or directing it too much turns it into little needles, a force of harm rather than of healing.

Exercise is potentially very helpful in strengthening your body against illness. Keep in mind, however, that strenuous, rough exercise (which builds up the larger muscles), tends to create blocks, whereas dancing, swimming, yoga, or tai chi all tend to balance and release the chakra flow.

Lemurian Chakra Healing

In Lemuria, a healer pulled energy from the patient's chakra relating to the illness, brought it into his or her body, turned it into positive energy and sent it back into the patient through a higher chakra. If, for example, the navel chakra reflected a problem, the healer would absorb energy from that point, heal it, then send it out the heart chakra to the patient's heart chakra and down to the navel area, replacing the energy. The key thing is to put energy back into the healed chakra, which otherwise could attract more illness; this also safeguards the healer against the illness.

Massage and Body Work

Massage and other body work are excellent for balancing energies throughout the body and allowing a proper chakra flow. It is difficult to relax and do a thorough job massaging your own body.

Samadhi

Samadhi is a Sanskrit word meaning evenness and describing a balance between inner body forces and forces from around the body. Seek Samadhi for a chakra that does not flow correctly. Sometimes breathing a flat breath—a breath that feels flat up and down the front of the chest—helps you bring in the sense of evenness. Filling the chakra with a lavender color may help, or you may simply ask to feel Samadhi. Working to feel Samadhi brings inner peace and quietude, facilitating growth and healing. When seeking Samadhi it is best to start with one of the heart chakras, moving on from there in whatever pattern you wish.

Rocks, Minerals, and Healing

Energies from rocks and minerals have a definite effect on chakras, bringing healing or awakening. Experiment with various rocks and minerals to see which attract you. Place them on different chakras and observe your energy responses. There are many books available on using crystals and minerals for healing or awakening chakras.

Radiance

It is difficult to maintain a healthy level. The body tends either to go into illness or weakness or into radiance; there has to be movement one way or the other. Radiance, meaning vitality and openness, is certainly preferable to illness, but to achieve it you must have good energy flow throughout your body. Think of the things that help you keep your body more radiantly alive. Your list might include exercise, diet, joy, smelling the flowers, love—all sorts of things. Keep a running list and add to it from time to time, and try to do something from your list on a daily basis. Eventually, you will naturally do what keeps you radiant.

Some useful books for rocks and minerals are:

Baer, Randall N. and Vicki Vittitow Baer. *Windows of Light*. New York: Harper and Row, 1984.

Fernie, William T., M.D. *The Occult and Curative Powers of Precious Stones*. New York: Rudolf Steiner Publications, 1973.

Gurudas. *Gem Elixers and Vibrational Healing*, Volumes I and II. San Raphael, CA: Cassandra Press, Vol. I, 1985, Vol. II, 1986.

Kunz, George Frederick. *The Curious Lore of Precious Stones*. Mineola, NY: Dover, 1970.

Raphaell, Katrina. *Crystal Healing*, Volume II. Santa Fe, NM: Aurora Press, 1987.

Chapter 13

Karma

Introduction

As above, so below.
Whatsoever ye sow, so shall ye reap.
For every action there is a reaction.
Voids must be filled.
All things change.
Give to receive.
Polarities will seek balance.

Karma is a Sanskrit word meaning "reaction follows action." It means that what you send out, you get back. Such a concept could scare people into not doing anything; "reactions" to errors might be too much to handle. But not to act when action is required for life and growth may bring as great a problem. Intuition is a great help in knowing when and when not to act or react. Relieve doubt, bring clarity and release the tensions which aggravate karma by filling yourself and the entire circumstance with love.

We tend to label unpleasant karma BAD and pleasant karma GOOD. Karma is actually neither good nor bad. It may be painful, but it also promotes growth. "Good karma" is used to describe a condition of good things; but the problem with desiring "good karma" is that you may put yourself in strange or difficult situations just so someone can pay you some "good karma" and get you out of it! Karma may not always be convenient, and to get caught up in doing good things for the sake of receiving good sometimes defeats the purpose. What karmic situations do is help people understand universal laws and how to work within their framework.

Learning the laws of karma and working within their framework, you lessen the possibility of creating more karma. Ego-attachments are almost certain to bring karma. We need to develop an attitude of detachment, which does not mean non-caring; a person may actually care more deeply and risk more while practicing detachment. The Old Testament concept of karma—"an eye for any eye, a tooth for a tooth"—is dated. More enlightened, we understand and work with the New Testament's message of forgiveness, which involves releasing karmic energies. Simply by understanding what you do, feel, or think, you release karmic energy. It is helpful to ask God, Jesus or a high spiritual master to facilitate this release.

We must change after karmic release, lest we bring similar experiences back upon ourselves, having not learned the lessons. The energy of lessons unlearned goes into the next opportunity for the lesson, by that time being more difficult.

Those who create karma may still be learning and evolving, but at a slower rate or on a lower path. Those who learn and use their energies correctly and are not caught up in attachment travel the higher, more spiritual path. The latter use more understanding and divine qualities in their interactions. In order to grow we must all go through learning experiences; our attitudes and feelings toward these experiences make the difference in how we travel the path. Not all problems, illness or misfortune should be labeled "karma." We are in an evolutionary process, periodically receiving new energies to work with, learn, and use, a process which strengthens our energies and our use of them. This then is not karma, but *opportunity*—to grow and develop.

Learning to tell the difference between karma and opportunity can change how you act or react to stimuli. Faced with opportunity, when a situation asks for growth and development, you will feel PUSHED to grow, explore, or try new things; you may have a sense of pioneering with your energies or going beyond what you thought you were capable of doing. But if the situation is karmic, you will feel confused and PULLED toward the action, as if you were part of a drama. You may not then or even later understand what is going on, so going with your intuitions is best. Some people psychically check into these situations to get information; others seek information from books or teachers. Whichever way is best for you, it is important to do your best with it and remember what you are learning. There are times when you have to learn completely new ways of doing things, so ask yourself: "How else can I handle this?" It may be the opposite of your habit. A leader may need to let others lead. A follower may need to take a leadership role.

Situational and Attitudinal Karma

There are two main types of personal karma: 1) situational, in which anything you have done to someone else in a past life is returned in kind to you by that person in this life; and 2) attitudinal karma, in which, for instance, all past life anger toward life or others affects all you do in this life.

Situational karma may go on for many lives; not till one person grows enough to want to change his or her actions or reactions, thus taking leave of the wheel of that interaction, will the dynamic cease.

Attitudinal karma attracts anger back, working likewise for fear and worry. You should become aware of all attitudes that are not in your best interest and work to release them. Filling yourself with love will cause all that you do to be filtered through love. A balance of good for all concerned is the best solution; work for "win-win" situations.

The Karma of Others

Most people get caught up in others' karma at one time or another. When we worry too much about others, or interfere where we shouldn't, we are caught. Instead of worrying, send blessings. It is the opinion of some that we should never do anything to interfere with another's karma. On the other side, there is the Christian attitude of helping to alleviate the karma or problems of others through healing, forgiveness of sins, walking the extra mile, sharing burdens and giving. I personally believe in the latter approach, but we should be careful not to meddle. There are many people who like to get involved in another's karma as a means of control or out of guilt; perhaps they are bored or fascinated by the other's concerns. Prayerful, intuitional consideration should influence your decision whether to get involved. Balance is important. Those whose Kundalini predominantly flows through the chakra at the back of the top of the head rather than through the crown tend not to interfere with others. Those whose Kundalini comes heavily out the front of the top of the head (seventh eye) tend to have an attitude of helping and living for others. For balance and direction, the main energy should flow out the crown chakra.

Group Karma

Groups may work on balance much as individuals. Determining for yourself the highest good of the group helps you decide on your level of involvement. Functioning from greater awareness, you will know whether to increase or decrease your interaction and will come to know the purpose of the karma. More than ever we need to be careful of group involvement. For some this challenge entails increased involvement; for others it means withdrawing into their own work.

Conscious Choice of Karma

Before we are born into a life we help make the decision of what karma we want to balance and in which areas we wish to grow. The more evolved a person is, the more choice he or she has in the planning. There are those who planned to release so much karma in this life as to be overwhelmed living through it; they have bitten off more than they can easily chew. Others may have ambitious plans for growth, or choose illness as a means of developing endurance, strength, understanding, and knowledge of illness. An illness may be part of a group's total growth; for instance, Helen Keller may have chosen her life as a way of demonstrating how the deaf and blind can function.

Karma's Positive Side

People may yearn to achieve certain goals they did not meet in a previous life, whether pertaining to relationships, career choices, growth and development, travel, artistic pursuit, or any other facet of life; the energy of the yearning has not been fulfilled and awaits an opportunity for completion. Everybody's choices are influenced to some extent by this karmic drive, fulfilling latent desires.

Chapter 14

Preparation for Voluntary Kundalini Release

Preparing for Release

It is possible to achieve several lifetimes of growth during one life by safely releasing, assimilating and using more Kundalini. Proper release requires time, patience and perseverance.

Once release is started, there is no turning back. It will continue on its own. Kundalini release is a process with its own intelligence and goal, blending with the spiritual at the crown chakra: The dance of shakti and shiva.

The more prepared your system, the easier the release and the faster the energies are assimilated to increase all levels of ability. Many people feel called to enter into this life but not all have qualified teachers to guide them. Many work with Kundalini who only have a sketchy knowledge of it. Most of the sources are Eastern; they are not always easily understood and are directed to those who dedicated their lives to spiritual growth. In the West we usually do not have the time (if it were even possible) to separate ourselves from life and concentrate on staying in the world and bringing the spiritual into it.

Many have been introduced into chakra work without exposure to the nadis, glands and the entire system. If chakra work is all you do, it is like concentrating on the wheels of a vehicle! Important, but what about the rest of it?

Caring for the physical body before, during and after Kundalini raising is very important; it is our living machine through which we express and receive. We achieve higher states of evolution only as our body permits; when the body denies us we feel encased or trapped in it. Instead of getting away from the body, we need to learn to bring it along. A transformed body feels great confidence, freedom and joy. (Chapter 2 suggests how to care for your body. If you doubt your body is adequate for further release, refer to those pages for further preparation.)

Exercises for Extra Kundalini Release

Revitalizing the Cells

Lie comfortably on your back. Do deep, peaceful breathing for a few minutes, then take several complete breaths. With your eyes closed, visualize a golden energy entering each cell and bringing new vitality. Then visualize *prana* coming in through the breath, traveling to each cell with the golden energy. Really FEEL this energy going into each cell.

Receiving Energies from the Universe

The earth is part of the universe and so is the recipient of its energies in all of their various frequencies. Meditate on this while doing deep, peaceful breathing. Ask the energies of the universe to balance the system, to modify excessive frequencies and bring needed ones. Visualize the energies becoming balanced. Also visualize becoming more open to the nutrients available in foods as well as in the universe. Energies you receive through food have been transmuted into the different frequencies necessary for your system. As the world's population continues to increase, it will be most beneficial to know how to use these energies directly instead of getting them transmuted through food. We already do this with the sun's vitamin D. People who receive their energies through breathing and absorbing the universe are called breatharians.

The physical body, as a living machine given to us for learning how to use energy and its different frequencies, is extremely important in our evolution. When we understand this fully, we will no longer need to be born in bodies; we will be able to use energy directly from the universe without the aid of a living machine (the body) transmuting energy into different frequencies for various purposes.

Rebuilding Cells

Vitamins and minerals are simply energy frequencies which the body needs for full development and function. When these needs are not met because of inadequate diet or the body's own inability to assimilate the energy from food, there need to be alternative ways. Some needs are met by inducing emotional or mental states of a frequency corresponding to the vitamin or mineral in which the body is deficient; but this is hard on the system, removing as much as it could possibly replace. Another method is to transmute a portion of excessive energy to the frequency needed to satisfy the deficiency; to do this well, however, you have to understand the frequencies and how to work with them. A third method is to pull the proper frequency into your system directly for the universe. *The first two methods are not recommended for beginners because of their difficulty.* The third is an excellent one to practice whether or not diet is adequate, raising the spiritual vibrations and training one to receive energies directly from the universe.

Stretching

This is one of the best and simplest exercises available. You should take time to stretch thoroughly before going to sleep, upon waking, and at various times during the day. Done prior to meditation, stretching unifies Self and Body, preparing it to assimilate knowledge later. It also releases blocks.

Cleansing the Head

Shake your head gently a few times, then slowly roll it around on your neck. Imagine or visualize it cleansed and refined by a shower of golden (Kundalini/mental) energy. (A silvery sheen would indicate more of a spiritual essence.) Alternate or at least balance these two colors so you do not develop lopsided. Follow this exercise by imagining the breath going up into your head, nourishing all the cells. Ideally, then, you would go outdoors and increase your vision in the psychic and spiritual areas of your brain by looking at the scenery or the horizon.

Releasing Blocked Areas

Contracting the Belly. This is for releasing the sexual, navel and solar plexus areas. Lie down supine on the floor and pull your knees to your chest so that the small of your back touches the floor. Tighten your belly muscles as much as possible from the pubic area to the rib cage and from side to side; then slowly lower your legs to a straight position without arching your back. Be sure your back and body are as relaxed as possible. Hold this muscle contraction while taking ten deep breaths. Move the energy from this area up and out the top of the head. Gradually do this exercise until you can hold the contraction for twenty breaths. This will release excess Kundalini from these areas, helping it on its way up the spine. It also helps conquer emotional states. Once each day is sufficient until the area feels cleansed; after that, do the exercise as the need arises.

Releasing the Chest Area. At times you may feel very depressed in the chest area, even to the point of feeling as if you are drowning, unable to cope with all the vibrations. The following exercise can alleviate this. Inhale and exhale deeply, expanding your entire chest cavity, front, back and sides. Visualize *prana* coming in with your breath, leaving through the skin to cover your entire body from the top of your head to your toes and fingers. Be sure your neck is relaxed. Let *prana* soothe the nerves of the skin.

Releasing the Neck Area. Find a comfortable position, holding your neck straight and your head as high and straight as is comfortable. Roll your tongue back into your mouth; hold there for five breaths, focusing your attention on the crown chakra. Let your neck be fully relaxed. Gradually increase the breaths until you can comfortably do fifteen. Once a day is sufficient until this area is cleansed, then do the exercise as the need arises.

Releasing the Glands. Kundalini and chakras affect the glands, excessive energy causing increased glandular activity and also physical problems, if the glands are blocked. For a variety of reasons, many people have blocked or tensed the areas around the glands, reducing their efficiency. The following exercise is designed to give you healthier, better functioning glands. Your first few times doing it you may be left feeling very heavy and tired, depending on the amount of energy released. Allow time for rest and open meditation afterwards. It is all right to do two or three areas at a time, but balance the energy overall so as not to create an overload. Once each week is enough for the entire system; later, do it only when you are blocked or you want to do it.

Visualize each gland in turn, beginning with the lower and ending with the pineal, as healthy and well-functioning, the surrounding area free from tensions and blocks. At the end of the exercise bathe the entire body in a golden light for a few minutes.

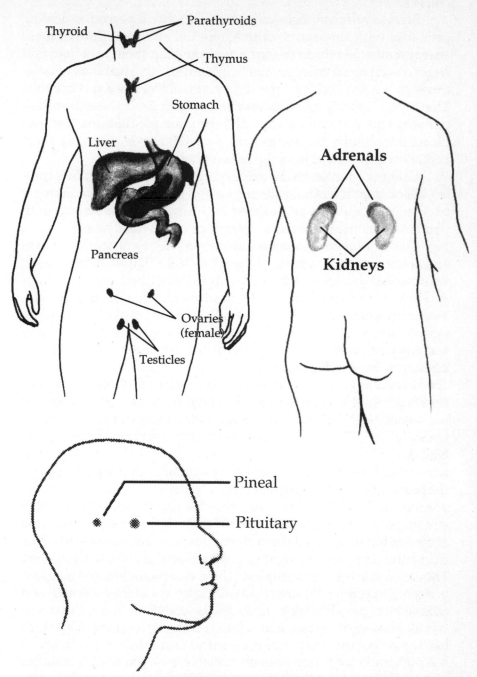

Locations of Organs and Glands.

Nerves

Nerves are extremely important whether a person is dealing primarily with spiritual or with Kundalini energies. Both of these energies manifest through the nerves, pushing them to extend and receive even more energy, thus heightening our awareness. Sometimes your nerves will feel raw, and you will feel tense and irritable. That is the time either to suspend or at least limit these exercises; perhaps you were doing so well with your meditations that you brought too much 220 energy into your 110 nerves. Calming them and allowing them to catch up is essential.

Calming Your Nerves. Imagine lying on a beach: The tide is coming in and gently washing all tension and negativity away, taking it back into the water to be cleansed in the ocean of life. Repeat until you have a calm and peaceful feeling all over your system.

Color Meditation. Sometimes your nerves lack or are deficient in one of the component parts of the white light. Think of the ends of your nerves all over your body; imagine them filled with a red light and love (love doesn't dig up old frustrations); then an orange light, a yellow light, a green light, blue light, and a purple light, ending with a radiant white light filling your nerve endings. Many times you will discover one of the colors rushing into the nerves; then you know you were deficient in it.

Visualizing. An excellent way to nourish and build up your nerves is to look at colors or visualize favorite ones. You may wish to use colored light bulbs to change the color energy of your area.

Nadis

Where your nerves power your physical body, the nadis power the higher mental and spiritual levels. Nadis are like nerve channels of a more subtle, etheric nature. There are many thousands of them and they are very important as vehicles for the entry and circulation of the life force (*prana*) in the system. This is an important part of the Kundalini experience, as *prana* releases and activates Kundalini. The Kundalini travels throughout these etheric nerves, refining and vivifying the entire system and availing you of higher spiritual and mental energies. The three main nadis (see Plate 3) are *Sushumna* (spiritual essence), which goes up the center of the spine; *Ida*, which has female polarity (negative in electrical terms); and *Pingala*, which has male polarity (positive in electrical terms). Ida and Pingala begin on either side of the base of the tailbone and weave back and forth around the spinal area (much as the snakes in the Caduceus of Hermes). They cross at the base of the skull, run over the top of the nose and end one at each corner of the nose.

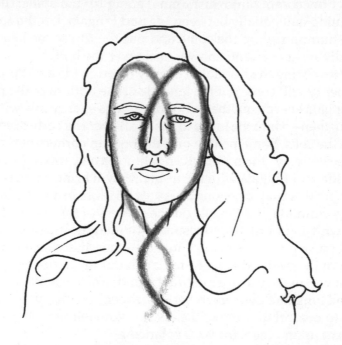

Closer view of Ida *&* Pingala *at corners of nose.*

In a good Kundalini release, the main force rises up Sushumna and the lesser forces rise up Ida and Pingala. When Ida receives an excessive release, you will experience an excess of energy in the emotional and intuitional bodies, leading to weepiness, a tendency to overeat, chills and difficulty staying warm, and getting caught in emotional and compassionate issues. When Pingala receives an excessive release, you may experience anomalies at the mental and will/spirit levels: hot flashes, sleeping problems, inability to eat, excessive mental pictures (usually of geometric shapes and lights), or psychic or spiritual sounds.

Balancing Exercises for Overloaded Ida or Pingala. Visualize the end of your tailbone (where Kundalini comes into Sushumna), free of stress and opened to receive the flowing Kundalini. Now visualize the bottom of the left side of the tailbone, where Ida begins, also opened and stress-free. Then visualize the bottom of the right side of the tailbone where Pingala begins, free of stress and gently opened. (If visualization is difficult for you, use your imagination, which the energy also follows). Visualize or imagine about half of the Kundalini flow coming into Sushumna, going up the spine; divide the remaining half equally between Ida and Pingala. Let the Kundalini in Sushumna rise up the spine and out the top of the head to mix with divine energy and shower back over the body.

Now bring the Kundalini energy through Ida and Pingala. The Ida energy will come out the left side of the bottom of the nose and the Pingala energy out the right side; let this energy mix with the in-breath, then go into the lungs to travel all over the body to refine and uplift the cells. Some people find the bottom corners of their noses itch excessively during this Kundalini release; mixing the energy from Ida and Pingala with the in-breath will bring some relief (five or six breaths may be enough). As a variation, bring the Kundalini energy from Ida and Pingala (at the corners of the nose) up into the head with an in-breath and visualize or imagine it cleansing and refining the inside of the head. You may either dissipate the excess energy out the nose exhaling or radiate it out the entire head.

If you make use of a qualified Kundalini teacher to balance the Ida and Pingala flow, remember it is imperative that you eventually learn to control and move the energy yourself so you are not dependent upon others for your balancing.

Massage. Full body massages release excess energy and contribute to a better balance and flow of energy.

Cleansing the Nadis. Find a comfortable position, preferably with your back and neck straight. Take deep, peaceful breaths for a few moments, then two complete breaths. Visualize the nadis, noting if any areas look dark or muddy. Fill yourself up with a silver sheen, letting all nadis be cleansed. Pay particular attention to Sushumna in the spine and Ida and Pingala alternating on either side of the spine.

Nadis Dance. Play background music of a tribal or belly-dance nature (this type of music promotes release of evolutionary energy.) Think of the superficial facia, the area just under your skin all over your body; let it feel alive and guide your dance. As you dance visualize or imagine the thousands of nadis all through your body glowing and silvery. Feel your evolutionary energy enlightened. Five or ten minutes may be all you want to do, as this dance is quite powerful. Follow the dance by lying down and entering an open, meditative state. To insure you are on a higher vibration, think of yourself as floating.

You may never feel totally ready, but don't hassle yourself; listen to your own urge to move along. You are the best judge of where you are. Trust yourself. After you've raised some Kundalini you can always go back to previous exercises for further work and there are plenty of other things you can do to enhance your overall development.

Chapter 15

Methods for Voluntary
Kundalini Release

WARNING

This chapter may be hazardous to the student's health. It is best to work with a qualified Kundalini teacher. I realize that this is not always possible and that some people will feel guided to release more energy on their own. But please exercise caution. You are dealing with very powerful energies.

By providing exercises for the unsupervised releasing of Kundalini I have probably opened myself to criticism from various sources. But with reasonable caution and common sense, many people can work alone. As mentioned before, the Aquarian Age is the time when information previously considered secret and available for the select few becomes available for all. In this new age the choice is, and should be, the individual's. Once you make the decision to go ahead and work for more releasing, do not be attached to it or fear it. Attachment and fear are forces that work against healthy release. Do not fear, but do respect the energy.

Having read the previous chapters and practiced the exercises, you may feel ready to release more Kundalini. If so, this chapter provides insights and exercises. BUT, if you are the kind of person who skips the first parts of books, including this one—if you have no intention of doing the exercises leading up to this point but just wanted to get into releasing more, let me caution you: *Take the time to read and study the previous chapters and do the exercises; otherwise you risk incurring problems, perhaps minor, perhaps traumatic.* Releasing more Kundalini is always something of a risk. If the exercises thus far have worked well and your life is on a fairly even keel, risk is minimized.

Kundalini is different in each person. You may not notice much change, or you may notice change after just one or two exercises; some people are more ready than others. If you have done a lot of cleansing, releasing new energy is faster and easier. *Those who have been on hard drugs may experience too much release in the beginning and should be extra cautious.* Some people are not at first aware of energy movement; this does not mean there is none. Wait before repeating an exercise until you are sure you have handled whatever you released.

When you are aware of what the energies feel like, and when you are able to move energy around, you stand a much better chance of controlling additional release. *Once released, there is no putting the energy back.* Released energy may affect you in one of three ways:

1/ it moves up the system, cleansing as it goes;

2/ it gets stuck in energy blocks for however long it takes to break through;

3/ it uses its own energy to turn back on itself; this is very unsafe and creates risk.

You may use the power of Kundalini to hold back the Kundalini itself for a period of time, but such a concentration of energy increases the risk of bodily harm.

Your Decision

Some exercises may not seem right for you. If an exercise does not feel right, do not do it. Everyone is different, and what works for one does not necessarily work for another. I have provided a variety of exercises so you have some choice. Take the time to re-read Chapter 2; many exercises contained therein are helpful after you have released more energy.

Never do the exercises on a full stomach; wait at least one hour after eating. Do not do the exercises when tired or just before doing something that will take a lot of concentration. Having done the exercises, you may be inclined to relive old illness; very vivid memories of illness may arise during cleansing. You may also relive old joys and traumas as they are released from your system. This does not mean you will be left with no memory of past experience; it only means the memory is being cleansed, thus releasing another energy block. The memory will remain, but its impact on life will be insignificant; it will simply be a part of the past.

You must keep faith in yourself and in the Divine while releasing. Sometimes, during deep Kundalini cleansings, it is possible to feel alienated from self, loved ones, society and God. Work for a balanced life and outlook during this period. Do not get caught in the experiences. Observe, but remain detached. This is much easier said than done, but try. It can be a great help if you have someone with whom to share your experience of Kundalini release, especially so when reliving traumatic experiences. Learning to work with the new energies is much like a child learning to handle and use the new body he or she has been given. Just don't become a bore with it. Find creative projects such as journaling or art work in order to use your new energy so it does not back up on you and become clogged in your system.

Possible Effects of Kundalini Release

Headaches and Other Pains

Most headaches are caused by blockages and concentrations of energy. If you seem to have too much energy in your head, let some go out the crown chakra and send the remainder down to your feet and let it go into the floor or ground. This is called grounding and is an excellent means of releasing energy concentrations. Also massage your head, as it tends to expand with Kundalini release.

Pain is a warning signal, a sign there is something wrong. If the problem appears to be an energy concentration or an improper flow in your body, lie down and fill the painful spot with a golden light; feel the energy equalize throughout your entire body. Or you may move the energy from the painful area to another area. If the pain seems to stem from lack of energy, send golden energy to it. If this does not work and the pain persists, stop all exercises. If the pain still persists, seek competent help from the outside. DO NOT WORK FOR KUNDALINI RELEASE IF YOU HAVE PAIN IN YOUR BODY; THIS COULD ONLY WORSEN THE PROBLEM.

During cleansing from Kundalini release, a current illness may become better or it may disappear. Many illnesses are caused by an excess of Kundalini blocked somewhere in the system wreaking havoc on the body. People on the spiritual path may encounter more illness if they have not learned to handle the extra energy released in their systems. The overload can surface as problems in any area of life.

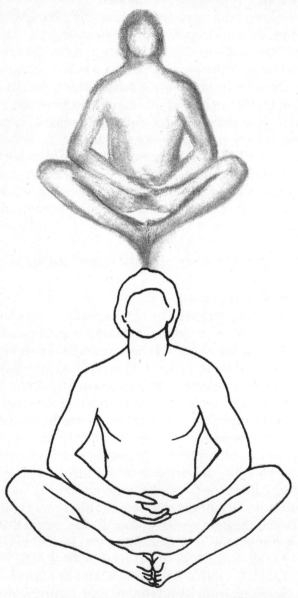

Out of body experiences are common with Kundalini release,
quite often through the crown chakra. There are other areas of the body
though which the travel is also accomplished.

Other Phenomena

During and after the exercises it is very likely any of a number of things will happen. You may experience out-of-body travel in full consciousness, or you may have memories of travel you made during sleep. Psychic gifts may appear or strengthen; they may also fade as other abilities appear. As your cleansing becomes more complete, your abilities come back stronger. Visual changes (such as seeing auras, pictures, and dots of light) will appear; in fact, at times, everything may appear as dots of light, geometric shapes, flames, vivid colors and forms. You may experience the nature sounds such as waterfalls, thunder, oceans, bees buzzing, and wind; or there may be musical sounds as if coming from the universe, including bells, flutes, violins, woodwinds, mighty orchestras or choruses. Sometimes you will also hear humming.

Observe and learn from all these things, but do not get caught in them. Remember the goal is the raising of the Kundalini and the joining of it with the divine energies for the ultimate in consciousness and awareness.

Preliminary Considerations

Bringing the Flow to the Spine

The Kundalini does not always feel hot traveling up the spine, especially when only small amounts are released. Some layers may bring chills to your system. Remember, outer layers have some heat, but the deepest layers have the intense heat. The Kundalini raising may feel like a lump moving up or just a pain. During exercises always continue to bring the energy up (think or visualize it going up) and be aware of its changes as it ascends; it may feel like an electric current, or a lightning streak, or there may be no sensations at all. If the latter, do not stop; if your awareness is not yet developed it is difficult to discern changes during the upward movement. Usually one does find some difference afterwards in the self or in attitudes.

If something happens to make it necessary to quit in the middle of an exercise, return to the exercise as soon as possible. If this is not possible, take just a moment and diffuse the energy throughout your body. NEVER LEAVE THE ENERGY IN ONE AREA. Always end a Kundalini releasing experience by mixing the Kundalini with the Divine and showering it over the body.

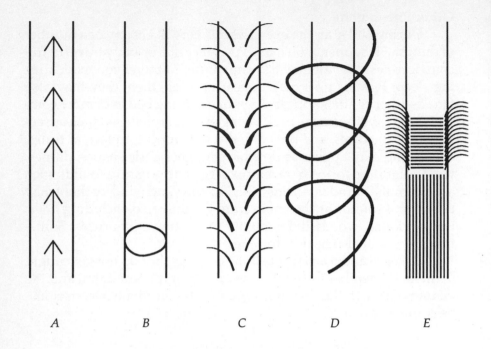

Kundalini travels up the spine in a variety of ways.
Some of the major ways shown above are as follows:

A—The ideal is to travel directly up the spine, sometimes it is quickly,
   and other times gently.
B—At times it feels like an egg.
C—The energy radiates out as it travels up.
D—If main channel is not open or clogged it may circle.
E—If the energy hits a strong block it will diffuse into body.

Wide Kundalini Raising

Sometimes people will experience spontaneous Kundalini release in a wide swath rather than in the narrow stream traveling
only up the spine. Such a raising is usually wide enough to go beyond the body limits and often forms a tube-like shape. The wide
raising can be much easier to handle than the narrow stream, as it
does not concentrate in one area. When a Kundalini rising produces
great pain, diffuse it by "thinking it" into the wide tube. Make sure
you bring it up above your head to mix with the divine energy for
the shower over your body.

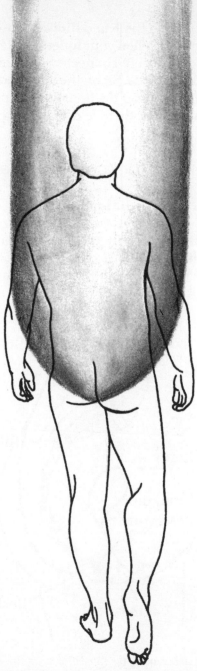

The wide Kundalini raising is sometimes spontaneous. It can release pressure when the body is depleted or blocked. It takes good mental control to direct it.

Relaxing a Tight Anal Area

People may impede the Kundalini's release by keeping their anal muscles very tense. When your inner or outer security is threatened, your anal area, closely connected with feelings of security, will be the first place to tense. Sit on the floor and lean back on your hands; raise your buttocks off the floor and drop them down again. Do this three or four times, then lie down and feel the area relaxed and at ease.

Methods for Kundalini Release

Mixing and Showering Technique
(To be used after all Kundalini releases)

Let the Kundalini mix with the Divine energy above the head and shower over the body (see Plate 4). As the energy comes into the body, visualize or imagine it going to cleanse and refine all of the cells.

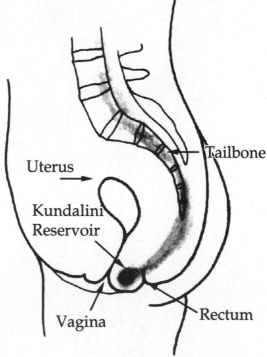

Alternately contracting and releasing the Kundalini reservoir can aid in the movement of the Kundalini up the spine. Some women who have released Kundalini incorrectly have severe menstrual problems, or uterine trouble, sometimes resulting in hysterectomies.

Basic Kundalini Release

Lie down with your back and neck straight (no pillow). (You may sit for this exercise, but our "western" backs are usually not strong enough to remain erect throughout the exercise; lying down precludes worrying about a straight back.) Concentrate on the area between your anus and genitals (the Kundalini reservoir, shown in the illustration). Tighten this area as much as possible and hold for five deep breaths. Then release for the count of five breaths. Repeat this sequence three times, then contract and release the area quickly ten times.

Visualize or imagine the Kundalini coming into the end of your spine and leaving out the top of your head as a wisp of grayish white, energy-like smoke. Finish by using the Mixing and Showering Technique above. Visualizing the energy as a wisp of smoke lessens the Kundalini released. If you think you have not released enough, you may repeat the raising part of the exercise several times. The grayish white color will soften power and is easier for your system to handle. Later you may wish to visualize or imagine the red-orange of the true Kundalini colors, or you may wish to transmute it into the radiant silver.

Rocking Release

Play background music during this exercise; belly dance or tribal music are particularly suitable for releasing evolutionary (Kundalini) energy. Sit on a thick pillow. Use the following rocking movements as they feel comfortable to you:

1/ back and forth;

2/ side to side;

3/ in a circular motion.

Visualize or imagine the Kundalini entering your spine, raising up and going out the top of your head. Complete the exercise, as always, with the Mixing and Showering Technique.

Rocking Release with a Partner. Follow the instructions given above with the addition of sitting back to back with your partner. As above, use thick pillows. Your buttocks should touch your partner's.

Release through Nadis

1/ Visualize Sushumna, Ida and Pingala (the three principal nadis) as pure and clean.

2/ Visualize or imagine the prana in Ida and Pingala going down to their source at either end of the bottom of the tailbone and then into the Kundalini reservoir between the anus and genitals. Hold it there and quiet your mind. After a few moments, release the energy.

3/ Visualize or imagine the prana in Sushumna (the spine) and let it drop into the reservoir. Hold it there for a few minutes with the mind quiet. After a few moments, release the energy.

4/ Inhale a deep breath, holding it in the heart area a moment as you visualize a red flame with it. Move the breath and the red flame back to the spine and down into the reservoir. Visualize the breath and flame setting fire to the latent Kundalini. Hold the breath for as long as possible and then release it.

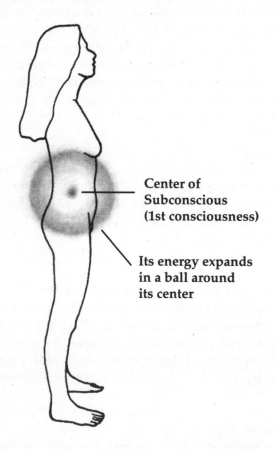

Center of Subconscious (1st consciousness)

Its energy expands in a ball around its center

The subconscious energy expands in a ball around its center.

Alternately tighten and release the Kundalini reservoir, forcing the Kundalini into the end of your spine, into Sushumna and up the spine and out the top of the head. Complete the exercise utilizing the Mixing and Showering Technique.

As a variation, visualize the combined energy going into the thousands of nadis, especially back into Ida and Pingala. Do not worry about where the nadis are; they are all over your body and thinking the energy into them will serve to find them. As another variation, do steps 1-4 in one sequence and continuing the exercise as listed.

First Consciousness (Subconscious) Exercise

Think of a spot approximately an inch behind and one inch below your navel; this is the area of the leyden cells, the center of the first consciousness. (There is also an area in the brain corresponding to the first consciousness, but the belly area is the true home).

Put your attention on the leyden cell area (see illustration). Breathe into it, feel the energy expand and let it drop down into the Kundalini reservoir. As the Kundalini releases, let it raise up through an imaginary tower about four inches in diameter beginning at the Kundalini reservoir and ending at the crown chakra. Complete the exercise with the Mixing and Showering Technique. As a variation, expand the energy in a large circle and rather than the four inch tower, do the wide release as explained above.

Puffing Exercise

From a standing position, slightly bend your knees so that the top of your body is slightly bent forward. Place your hands at your hips and with mouth closed begin to huff and puff like a steam locomotive pulling its load up a hill, letting your solar plexus and belly area move in and out. Visualize the Kundalini being pulled up the hill—up your spine. Do this only about six times in the beginning; work up to twenty times. As always, complete the exercise with the Mixing and Showering Technique.

As a variation, move the energy around the brains for cleansing and refining before releasing it out of the crown chakra; you may wish to visualize a golden-colored energy. Another variation (only use if you have strong mental control of the energy) is to drop the sexual energy into the Kundalini reservoir and bring the combination up the spine and out through the crown chakra.

Maithuna

Tantric Yoga has a ritual for the Kundalini release through sexual union, called maithuna, involving elaborate preparations, extensive training and a detailed ritual. Its purpose is to heighten the sexual feelings so that the energy becomes sufficiently strong and intense to awaken the Kundalini.

Sexual climaxes are not allowed in the practice of maithuna. Instead, you are to sublimate the energy into the Kundalini or spiritual experience, thus awakening the Kundalini and helping it reach the crown chakra for a spiritual awakening. Much control is required to "force the energy up the spine" and keep from climaxing.

It is possible to do this exercise without the elaborate preparations and training of the classical maithuna experience. But you are still obliged to treat it as any other Kundalini raising experience in this book; you must first prepare and cleanse your system.

Westerners may find it more helpful to end with climaxing so that the lower abdominal area does not become too clogged with energies, which can easily happen when there is a heightening of sexual energies and no adequate release.

First, begin with a willing partner; discuss any necessary preparations or rituals. Make up the rituals; include candles, incense, music or whatever is appropriate. Plan the time and place so you will be undisturbed. Massage, meditation on Kundalini raising, or breathing exercises may be a part of the preparation. There may be love play both before and during maithuna union. The usual position (others may also be used) is for the man to sit down with legs outstretched. The woman then sits astride the man facing him. They both then entwine their legs around each other. Movement is then used only to heighten the sensations and increase the passion, while still holding back climax. When you are both highly sexually aroused, let the energy drop down into the Kundalini reservoir at the end of the spine. Focus your attention in the Kundalini reservoir and gently massage each other's spine and crown chakra. Then with your arms around each other, but your backs and heads straight, put your awareness about three inches above your heads. Keep your minds still and your awareness open. Move the energy up your spines and through the crown chakras. Complete the exercise with the Mixing and Showering technique.

After finishing the exercise, lie down side by side, touching. Be in open meditation for at least twenty minutes to allow for messages and insights to appear. Share the experiences. (If you desire a climax, it can come either before or after meditation).

Now you can take a water shower!

Spiritual Light

Visualize or imagine a ball of white light approximately two feet in diameter resting above your head. Slowly bring it down into your head, awakening and developing the head in general, but the pineal gland in particular. After a few minutes, bring the ball of light slowly down through your body, the center of the ball going through the spine. Take it all the way to the Kundalini reservoir and feel the union of spiritual and Kundalini energies (see illustration on page 184). Bring this combination into your tailbone, up the spine and out the crown chakra. Since the energies are already mixed, complete the exercise simply with the showering technique.

Candle Flame

The Kundalini, flowing in the normal manner, resembles a candle flame, everflowing and gentle. When large amounts are released it is like the wind blowing the flame longer and larger. Visualize or imagine the Kundalini reservoir as a candle. Let feelings of Divine love light the candle. Watch the flame as it goes up the spine and out the crown chakra. Complete with the Mixing and Showering Technique. As a variation, see the showering of energy as sparks of light (see Plate 5); or, after the showering, feel the Kundalini in your system as a softly glowing candle.

Cautions

1/ Don't try to do all of these exercises at once; you will release too much.

2/ Wait at least a week or two between exercises in order to assimilate the energies released and make them useable.

3/ If you find yourself getting excessively hyper or unable to cope well with everyday demands, wait until you feel more capable of handling extra energy before continuing.

4/ If the Kundalini stays stuck in your spine, lie down on the floor with a crystal above your head and pointing away from your head. The power of the crystal will help move the energy. A multi- or double-terminated crystal is best.

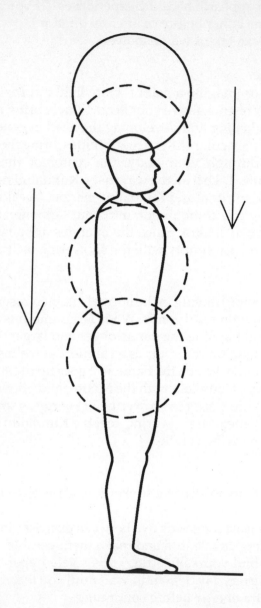

Visualize or image a white ball of light coming from above your head down into your body. Bring it into the Kundalini reservoir to release Kundalini. Take the combination back up and out the top of your head.

Doing Your Best

To make the best use of the new energy, spend a part of each day with spiritual thoughts, affirmations, or reading spiritual texts. When these practices seem very alien is when they are most needed. During Kundalini cleansing and releasing periods it is also an excellent idea to reflect on new possibilities, as Kundalini brings new abilities and gifts. Practice using the new talents. It is a new life, with the blessing of the Shakti-Shiva union. Make the most of it!

Chapter 16

Attributes of Enlightenment

ENLIGHTENMENT: to be filled with light, to comprehend the light, to know the light, to function from the light; to have the light on all knowledge and to radiate the light.

In an enlightened state, all senses are heightened so much that they scarcely seem to be related to our ordinary senses. For instance, trees, flowers or rocks might appear radiant and velvety; you will see their energy and feel their presence and their awareness of you. You will feel like you share a very deep connection.

- You will be able to see other people's glowing, luminous higher energies, even when the darker human energies are prevalent in their force fields.

- You will be able to change focus, see into other dimensions, converse with the beings who live there.

- You will be able to see energies manifesting and know what they will become. You will also be able to see different frequencies of energy with their varied forms.

- You will have an understanding of the universal laws and how to operate within their framework. You will have insight into the various religions and how they have interpreted the laws. You will feel parareligious and paraphilosophical, aware of all levels of truths.

- You will be filled with constant joy or bliss (although you may also have feelings of sadness or grief in particular situations).

- You will have genius level abilities and great artistic and creative abilities.

- You will have a deep sense of oneness with other humans, animals and all nature, a deep sense of connectedness with the Creator and the cosmos.

- You will have great powers and full understanding of how to use them. Some of the powers or gifts include: walking in the air or on water, levitation, ability to be invisible in a crowd, ability to generate enough body heat to melt a snow-field, command over the environment; healing, speaking in tongues, casting out devils; imperviousness to poisons; wise or inspired speech; heightened senses, such as clairvoyance, clairaudience, clairsentience, awareness of the past, present and future events; and the greatest power of all—love, all consuming, all forgiving, unconditional, LOVE.

As you go through the Kundalini process toward enlightenment, some of these gifts will come and go. The amount of ability you have will depend on the amount of Kundalini flowing and useable at the time. Do not get caught up in receiving the gifts and powers; they will come when your main attention is focused on the enlightenment (or the Kingdom of Heaven, as it is termed in Christianity). Focusing on the powers may actually slow you down.

Gopi Krishna's writings will give you a deeper understanding of this process as it functions in the Aquarian Age. Ancient texts will give you background and foundation.

Samadhi Exercise

The following exercises are based on "Samadhi," a Sanskrit term meaning "evenness" (a perfect balance) which describes a contemplative, almost trance-like state that helps you develop the higher attributes of consciousness.

Lower Samadhi. Lower Samadhi has seven attributes. Using color—the lightest pastels, shimmering on a transparent light background—can help access the levels.

Lying down, enter a contemplative state, that is, being one with what you are contemplating. Because of the power, three to five minutes on each color is plenty.

Lavender/healing, psychic heat. Feel yourself filled with the lightest of lavenders shimmering on a transparent light background. Meditate on its attributes. Now think the energy of the color into a psychic heat (tumo). Feel yourself coming into alignment with the true nature of self. Do each color in turn, meditating on the corresponding attributes:

Light blue/bliss, devotion; be engulfed by it.

Light green/experiencing or knowing; what do you experience or know?

Light yellow/cosmic consciousness; what mental perceptions did you have?

Light melon (light muskmelon)/power; feel the peacefulness of it.

Light rose/all consuming, all pervading love; be engulfed by it.

Light pink (a variation of light rose)/creativity; feel changes emerging.

Radiant Light/oneness with all; be engulfed by it.

Variation of the Lower Samadhi. Think of each color and its attributes one at a time. Bring the pastel color into its jewel tone, the shade of action. Meditate on how you would like to act (bring into manifestation) the attribute of the color.

Lavender/into amethyst;

Blue/into sapphire;

Green/into emerald;

Yellow/into yellow citrine;

Orange/into orange carnelian;

Rose/into ruby;

Pink/into pink tourmaline;

Radiant Light/into diamond.

Unless you have lots of time to deal with the energies the Radiant Light exercise will release, you may wish to do the exercise with only one color per day.

Higher Samadhi. Higher Samadhi has the highest bliss or devotion; in it, nothing else exists. It has a feeling of unmanifested energy or a void. Fill yourself completely with bliss or devotion (whichever word is best for you). Breathe into it, float, be immersed in it.

All senses lead to the Divine. Learn to find the Divine (the ultimate) in your senses of touch, smell, hearing, taste, and sight. For example, smell a rose (or imagine it) until you reach a higher level or oneness with the rose and with God.

The ultimate desire is for enlightenment. Each time you desire something, meditate on how it could bring you closer to enlightenment. Is it symbolic of a deeper desire?

As you develop, you will find spontaneous exercises coming to your consciousness. Do take the time to do them; write down what they are and your results. The higher you evolve, the more aware you will be of what you need to work on from within your system.

Chapter 17

The Holy Spirit and Kundalini

Until recent years, little has been known about Kundalini in the Western cultures. Many Westerners have thought that this concept was only a part of Eastern religions, but this energy is universal and has always operated within human beings whether or not they had active knowledge of the process. Christian mystics describe experiences in their writings which closely resemble the effects of Kundalini. They attributed these manifestations to the work of the Holy Spirit, and in a sense this is true, as the Holy Spirit can indeed release the Kundalini energy.

There are vast differences between the Kundalini energy and the energy of the Holy Spirit. Kundalini is an evolutionary energy and is of the Earth. All people have some Kundalini flowing, leading to the development of mind-knowledge and power. The energy of the Holy Spirit, on the other hand, is a divine energy of God leading to the development of love and wisdom. The ultimate goal of Kundalini is enlightenment and the ultimate goal of the Christian is to be one with or filled with God and/or Christ; whichever we call it, it is the same goal.

Some people choose a path primarily of faith and devotion, others one of knowledge and practice. We might make the distinction that Kundalini relates to the mind of God and the Holy Spirit relates to the heart of God.

The most interesting result of the advanced stages of any path is that, regardless of path, in the higher stages of growth each person begins to develop in a similar way. A person concentrating on the mental path will develop more of the love/wisdom through expansion into oneness and the practice of compassion, while the person devoted to love/wisdom will develop more of the knowledge/ power through understanding and controlling the process. All of us are ultimately called to develop both areas.

Many in Eastern religions have searched for enlightenment or God primarily through understanding the power of Kundalini, how it works, how to raise it, and what it does in human evolution. There is a lot of knowledge about it, although it is hidden in symbolic language. Yogis who have reached advanced stages of raising and developing their Kundalini attain the great paranormal powers called "siddhis." They have learned how to change energies and use them to accomplish certain purposes. Christian mystics, on the other hand, probably had very little knowledge of the process, yet through the workings of the Holy Spirit attained enlightenment. These mystics have been able to perform paranormal feats called "miracles." Faith in God replaced the understanding of how the miracles happened. Both yogis and mystics suffered and endured many things on account of their goals. Dedication and a willingness to do whatever was necessary seem to be characteristics of both.

Modern-day searchers are looking at various paths, including Christian, Buddhist, Hindu, Jewish, American Indian, Rosicrusion, Sufi, and ancient Egyptian. You do not have to give up your basic beliefs. In fact, studying other religions sometimes helps you understand your own religious beliefs better.

If traditional religions are to keep pace with the deepening spiritual interest of humanity, however, the time seems ripe for a renewal within the systems. There is a growing hunger for the mystical path and the knowledge of the mysteries of God which has not been totally satisfied by the current programs within our churches. Often, for the individual who longs to feel God's love and God's presence in his or her life, the rules, regulations and old attitudes are stifling. The desire to be both spiritual and human—to open awareness of our spirit and of our human potential—is the motivating drive behind this blending of paths.

It is time for modern-day searchers to take their own needs for development into account in both the spiritual and human realms. They need to find a common ground leading to an understanding of the process and to ultimate enlightenment. We must develop a new vocabulary. The mystical language of any path contains such deep symbolism that it is usually totally comprehensible only to those who have had similar experiences. New vocabulary brings new understanding, which helps us discern the relevance of old truths.

An example of a vocabulary problem is in the use of the word "sin." Many people do not comprehend what "sin" really means in their lives; what seems sinful to one generation does not to another, or the degree of sinfulness seems to change. Sometimes sin refers only to overt acts, and sometimes to each unholy thought. Another source of confusion is when religious groups alter their doctrines and call something acceptable which they previously considered a sin; then the question arises: is the sin committed against the church or against God? Did the church change its mind or did God? Such questions have caused people to seriously question the doctrines of their religions. They wonder whether their spiritual growth is between themselves and God or between themselves and a particular faith and its doctrines. These questions are deeply troubling. Many sincere people have left the organized, traditional religions in search of greater personal understanding of their connections with the Divine source.

One way of resolving the confusion is to examine the concept of sin through the use of the word "karma," a Sanskrit term meaning "reaction follows action." People are beginning to discover that all of life needs to be accounted for, not just particular actions called "sins," and that Christ and high spiritual masters are able to transmute all "negative" or inappropriate behavior into good or positive energy. We need both areas of growth: spiritual and mental, Holy Spirit and Kundalini. We may accelerate our growth and shorten the time we need to attain enlightenment and that total Christ-like love by integrating these two avenues. For the first time in history, the knowledge of many paths is available for the dedicated seeker.

Chapter 18

Kundalini in the Future

Values

One of the greatest values of the union of Kundalini and spiritual energies—Shakti and Shiva, female with male—is a deepened awareness of the cosmos. It takes a person out of the narrow, individualistic lifestyle so prevalent today. A person who is refined and cleansed by the Kundalini and spiritual energies has much less desire to make life complicated and experiences a natural drive back to the basics of living more simply. The result is a richly content personal and inner life and less reliance upon material and social structures. People become more interested in empowering others, thus sharing power rather than taking all they can get.

In the past, most enlightened people were inclined to retreat from the world; the games of living had no meaning for them any longer. But the energies of the Aquarian Age have helped the enlightened take a more active part in the guidance of the human race through government, education, healing and other progress-oriented fields. The spiritual areas will continue to need the guidance of the enlightened, as the salvation of humankind depends on bringing a spiritual and cosmic awareness into all of life. With a cosmic understanding of life and balance, there would need be no air, water, or earth pollution, nor destructive activity in general.

Need for Adequate Education

Kundalini awakening is not a "gimmick." It is not the latest fad or something in which only strange people in isolated retreat centers "indulge." It should be researched and studied by all, so that the best use of Kundalini energy and awakening is understood and open to everyone. It is imperative that people familiarize themselves with this power. It is also imperative that some people be trained in Kundalini therapy; there is already a need for this. Too much of today's counseling is for the effect of the problem and not the cause. Improper energy flow is the cause of many emotional and mental problems. Neurotic or psychotic behavior is the effect. When people are trained to develop more viable energy patterns and flows, they can avoid getting caught in emotional and mental conflicts.

Children now receive physical education in schools; health checkups are required and counseling is, many times, provided as need arises. But the Kundalini approach has more to do with total training and education for life. Kundalini checkups would be a valuable part of a child's education. Specialists, trained in a knowledge of where the Kundalini is blocked or concentrated in a person, could spot potential criminals, potential sexual perverts and others with unhealthy outlooks on life, and suggest therapy early on.

Kundalini tests could also indicate the child who is a potential genius, or the one who appears retarded but is actually held back by blocked energies. Periodic checks or tests could determine if a child was making the best use of the energy in terms of its direction and flow.

At this point, the possibilities of Kundalini tests and therapy as aids to growth and development of our children can only be imagined. The opportunities seem tremendous. Methods would have to be developed and people would have to be trained in their use. It would probably be through private schools or private practice that such Kundalini therapy first becomes available. Many criminals, seemingly otherwise well-adjusted, have stated they do not know why they did what they did. Energy that has been concentrated or blocked for too long a time tends to "explode," much as a pressure cooker would explode if there were no release. When this energy gets out of control it can take over, increase any kind of feeling or thought, perhaps even causing a person to be temporarily insane.

There are people whose long-term mental problems were caused by improper Kundalini flow, people who could be cured by Kundalini therapy with a qualified Kundalini therapist.

Retreat or Involvement

In India and other countries it has been the practice of people interested in the development of Kundalini to leave the daily life of family, friends and work and enter an ashram or temple. They retreat from life as they know it and begin a new life where the atmosphere is conducive to growth, with people who have similar goals to guide them. But in the Aquarian Age and in this country things are very different. Very few people can afford the luxury of setting themselves apart for study when the inner urge arises. Those who do feel a need to retreat may not want their families to suffer the hardship their leaving would cause. It is a time in our human history when people should, in most cases, continue with their daily lives as a part of society, but still work on inner growth. This is much more difficult in some ways; in others it is much more rewarding, as growth and development then become a part of a total life. There will still be those who are able to separate themselves from society and work on their growth. Re-entry into society is not particularly easy for them; they may experience a total break with society as they knew it.

There will be more centers and retreat areas available to provide Kundalini therapy and education for shorter periods of time. It will be a part of our new growth field, a field that has become a very important part of our culture.

Regardless of how you choose to work with your Kundalini, you must always remember that the responsibility for it remains yours. You cannot delegate the responsibility to a guru or leader. It is wise to learn from others, but foolish to give up responsibility for yourself.

We Are Not Alone

While most of the benefits of Kundalini work discussed in this book have been related to the individual, the individual is not the only benefactor. Society and the world benefit by each individual's growth, no matter how small or great. As one person grows, so do others; as one person blocks growth, so are others held back. If enough specks of dirt are put into a pail of clean water, mud will result. The same is true of negativity: the more negativity introduced into life, no matter what the sources, the muddier life will become. But the more enlightenment that occurs in the world, the more we will each see clearly and thus increase our own enlightenment.

No one is alone in growth. Nor is the world alone. What happens on this earth causes energy of different manifestations to reach out into the cosmos.

People talk about peace without really understanding what it can be. It is not just the absence of war or disagreements. More truthfully, it is allowing the cosmic flow of the Creator to flow through everyone, working for total harmony and joy. It is possible to have inner peace during war, disagreements or other tragedies of life. The more that people have inner peace, the more harmoniously they will settle disputes. This is one of the gifts of the union of the energies—inner peace.

Conclusion

Kundalini release cannot be lightly dismissed for much longer. Aquarian Age energies are causing it to move in most people to some degree, bringing about a search for the spiritual side of life, more generally causing a movement for a "holistic" view or approach to life. The more everyone understands this tremendous force and its implication in individuals as well as the total life of the planet, the more easily and quickly will we all reap its benefits.

Selected Glossary

Atma
Great Self.

Brahman
Expansion. Evolution. The Absolute. Creator. Preserver. Destroyer of the Universe.

Chakra
(Skt) "Wheel." One of many energy vortices on our etheric body (q.v.).

Contemplative State
A condition in which you are one with that which you are contemplating.

Ida
One of the three main nadis. Female Polarity.

Karma
(Skt) "Reaction follows action." What you send out, you get back.

Kundalini
(Skt) "Circular Power." An individual's basic evolutionary force. The dormant, innate powers of divinity within an individual, personified as the sleeping Goddess Kundalini.

Kundalini Reservoir
Where the dormant Kundalini awaits, located at the base of the spine.

Maithuna
A ritual for Kundalini release through sexual union. From Tantric Yoga.

Mantra
(Skt) "Sacred counsel. Formula." Thought form. A mystical formula for invocation.

Nadi
Where your nerves power your physical body, the nadis power your higher mental and spiritual levels.

Pingala
One of the three main nadis. Male polarity.

Prana
Life-force.

Samadhi
(Skt) "Evenness." A perfect balance. A contemplative, almost trance-like state that helps you develop the higher attributes of consciousness.

Siddhis
Great paranormal powers to change and use energy for certain purposes, attained by yogis who have reached advanced stages of raising and developing their Kundalini.

Shakta Yoga
Energy discipline. The Divine spark of life force.

Sushumna
One of the three main nadis. Spiritual essence.

Tai Chi
An ancient Chinese form of energy movement, very effective in releasing and moving energy.

Tumo
Psychic heat.

STAY IN TOUCH

On the following pages you will find listed, with their current prices, some of the books now available on related subjects. Your book dealer stocks most of these and will stock new titles in the Llewellyn series as they become available. We urge your patronage.

To obtain our full catalog, to keep informed about new titles as they are released and to benefit from informative articles and helpful news, you are invited to write for our bimonthly news magazine/catalog, *Llewellyn's New Worlds of Mind and Spirit*. A sample copy is free, and it will continue coming to you at no cost as long as you are an active mail customer. Or you may subscribe for just $10.00 in the U.S.A. and Canada ($20.00 overseas, first class mail). Many bookstores also have *New Worlds* available to their customers. Ask for it.

Stay in touch! In *New Worlds'* pages you will find news and features about new books, tapes and services, announcements of meetings and seminars, articles helpful to our readers, news of authors, products and services, special money-making opportunities, and much more.

Llewellyn's New Worlds of Mind and Spirit
P.O. Box 64383-592, St. Paul, MN 55164-0383, U.S.A.
* * *

TO ORDER BOOKS AND TAPES

If your book dealer does not have the books described on the following pages readily available, you may order them directly from the publisher by sending full price in U.S. funds, plus $3.00 for postage and handling for orders *under* $10.00; $4.00 for orders *over* $10.00. There are no postage and handling charges for orders over $50.00. Postage and handling rates are subject to change. UPS Delivery: We ship UPS whenever possible. Delivery guaranteed. Provide your street address as UPS does not deliver to P.O. Boxes. Allow 4-6 weeks for delivery. UPS to Canada requires a $50.00 minimum order. Orders outside the U.S.A. and Canada: Airmail—add retail price of book; add $5.00 for each non-book item (tapes, etc.); add $1.00 per item for surface mail.

FOR GROUP STUDY AND PURCHASE

Because there is a great deal of interest in group discussion and study of the subject matter of this book, we feel that we should encourage the adoption and use of this particular book by such groups by offering a special quantity price to group leaders or agents.

Our special quantity price for a minimum order of five copies of *Kundalini and the Chakras* is $38.85 cash-with-order. This price includes postage and handling within the United States. Minnesota residents must add 6.5% sales tax. For additional quantities, please order in multiples of five. For Canadian and foreign orders, add postage and handling charges as above. Credit card (VISA, MasterCard, American Express) orders are accepted. Charge card orders only ($15.00 minimum order) may be phoned in free within the U.S.A. or Canada by dialing 1-800-THE-MOON. For customer service, call 1-612-291-1970. Mail orders to:

LLEWELLYN PUBLICATIONS
P.O. Box 64383-592, St. Paul, MN 55164-0383, U.S.A.

Prices subject to change without notice.

WHEELS OF LIFE: A User's Guide to the Chakra System
by Anodea Judith

An instruction manual for owning and operating the inner gears that run the machinery of our lives. Written in a practical, down-to-earth style, the fully-illustrated book will take the reader on a journey through aspects of consciousness, from the bodily instincts of survival to the processing of deep thoughts.

Discover this ancient metaphysical system under the new light of popular Western metaphors—quantum physics, elemental magick, Kabalah, physical exercises, poetic meditations, and visionary art. Learn how to open these centers in yourself, and see how the chakras shed light on the present world crises we face today. And learn what you can do about it!

This book will be a vital resource for: Magicians, Witches, Pagans, Mystics, Yoga Practitioners, Martial Arts people, Psychologists, Medical people, and all those who are concerned with holistic growth techniques.

The modern picture of the Chakras was introduced to the West largely in the context of Hatha and Kundalini Yoga and through the Theosophical writings of Leadbeater and Besant. But the Chakra system is equally innate to Western Magick: all psychic development, spiritual growth, and practical attainment is fully dependent upon the opening of the Chakras!

0-87542-320-5, 6 x 9, 520 pgs., softcover, illus.   **$14.95**

ECSTACY THROUGH TANTRA
by John Mumford

This beautifully illustrated book gives you the information on Tantra that has long been hidden. It is written by one of the world's foremost experts in the ancient art of Tantra and is very understandable to the novice.

Dr. Mumford guides the reader through mental and physical exercises aimed at developing psychosexual power; he details the various sexual practices and positions that facilitate "psychic short-circuiting" and the arousal of Kundalini, the Goddess of Life within the body. He shows the fundamental unity of Tantra with Western Wicca, and he plumbs the depths of Western sex magick, showing how its techniques culminate in spiritual illumination.

It includes a special section on a Tantric weekend, taking the reader through the actual process. Color plates, airbrush paintings and wonderful temple photos abound.

0-87542-494-5, 162 pgs., 6 x 9, color plates, illus., softcover   **$12.95**

CRYSTAL HEALING: The Next Step
by Phyllis Galde

Discover the further secrets of quartz crystal! Now modern research and use shows that crystals have even more healing and therapeutic properties than had been previously realized. Learn why polished, smoothed crystal is better to use to heighten your intuition, improve creativity and for healing.

Learn to use crystals for reprogramming your subconscious to eliminate problems and negative attitudes that prevent success. Here are techniques that people have successfully used—not just theories.

This book reveals newly discovered abilities of crystals now accessible to all, and is a sensible approach to crystal use. *Crystal Healing* will be your guide to improve the quality of your life and expand your consciousness.

0-87542-246-2, 224 pgs., illus., mass market   **$3.95**

CHAKRA THERAPY
by Keith Sherwood

This is an excellent how-to book on healing. Sherwood's previous book, *The Art of Spiritual Healing*, has helped many people learn how to heal themselves and others. *Chakra Therapy* follows in the same direction: Understand yourself, know how your body and mind function and learn how to overcome negative programming so that you can become a free, healthy, self-fulfilled human being.

This book fills in the missing pieces of the human anatomy system left out by orthodox psychological models. It serves as a superb workbook. Within its pages are exercises and techniques designed to increase your level of energy, to transmute unhealthy frequencies of energy into healthy ones, to bring you back into balance and harmony with your self, your loved ones and the multidimensional world you live in. Finally, it will help bring you back into union with the universal field of energy and consciousness.

Chakra Therapy will teach you how to heal yourself by healing your energy system because it is actually energy in its myriad forms which determines a person's physical health, emotional health, mental health and level of consciousness.

0-87542-721-9, 270 pgs., 5-1/4 x 8, illus., softcover   **$7.95**

THE ART OF SPIRITUAL HEALING
by Keith Sherwood

Each of you has the potential to be a healer; to heal yourself and to become a channel for healing others. Healing energy is always flowing through you. Learn how to recognize and tap this incredible energy source. You do not need to be a victim of disease or poor health. Rid yourself of negativity and become a channel for positive healing.

Become acquainted with your three auras and learn how to recognize problems and heal them on a higher level before they become manifested in the physical body as disease.

Special techniques make this book a "breakthrough" to healing power, but you are also given a concise, easy-to-follow regimen of good health to follow in order to maintain a superior state of being.

0-87542-720-0, 224 pgs., 5-1/4 x 8, illus., softcover   **$7.95**

THE INNER WORLD OF FITNESS
by Melita Denning

Because the artificialities and the daily hassles of routine living tend to turn our attention from the real values, *The Inner World of Fitness* leads us back by means of those natural factors in life which remain to us: air, water, sunlight, the food we eat, the world of nature, meditation, sexual love and the power of our own wishes—so that through these things we can re-link ourselves in awareness to the great non-material forces of life and of being which underlie them.

The unity and interaction of inner and outer, keeping body and psyche open to the great currents of life and of the natural forces, is seen as the essential secret of youthfulness and hence of radiant fitness. Regardless of our physical age, so long as we are within the flow of these great currents, we have the vital quality of youthfulness: but if we begin to close off or turn away from those contacts, in the same measure we begin to lose youthfulness.

0-87542-165-2, 240 pgs., 5-1/4 x 8, illus., softcover   **$7.95**

16 STEPS TO HEALTH AND ENERGY:
A Program of Color & Visual Meditation, Movement & Chakra Balance
by Pauline Wills and Theo. Gimbel

Before an illness reaches your physical body, it has already been in your *auric* body for days, weeks, even months. By the time you *feel* sick, something in your life has been out of balance for a while. But why wait to get sick to get healthy? Follow the step-by-step techniques in *16 Steps to Health and Energy*, and you will open up the energy circuits of your subtle body so you are better able to stay balanced and vital in our highly toxic and stressful world.

Our subtle anatomy includes the "energy" body of seven chakras that radiate the seven colors of the spectrum. Each chakra responds well to a particular combination of yoga postures and color visualizations, all of which are provided in this book.

At the end of the book is a series of sixteen "workshops" that helps you to travel through progressive stages of consciousness expansion and self-transformation. Each session deals with a particular color and all of its associated meditations, visualizations and yoga postures. Here is a truly holistic route to health at all levels! Includes sixteen color plates.

0-87542-871-1, 224 pgs., 6 x 9, illus., softcover   **$12.95**

THE WOMEN'S BOOK OF HEALING
by Diane Stein

At the front of the women's spirituality movement with her previous books, Diane Stein now helps women (and men) reclaim their natural right to be healers. Included are exercises which can help you to become a healer! Learn about the uses of color, vibration, crystals and gems for healing. Learn about the auric energy field and the Chakras.

The book teaches alternative healing theory and techniques and combines them with crystal and gemstone healing, laying on of stones, psychic healing, laying on of hands, chakra work and aura work, color therapy. It teaches beginning theory in the aura, chakras, colors, creative visualization, meditation, health theory and ethics with some quantum theory. Clear quartz crystals and 46 gemstones are discussed in detail, arranged by chakras and colors.

The Women's Book of Healing is a book designed to teach basic healing (Part I) and healing with crystals and gemstones (Part II). Part I discusses the aura and four bodies; the chakras; basic healing skills of creative visualization, meditation and color work; psychic healing; and laying on of hands. Part II begins with a chapter on clear quartz crystal, then enters gemstone work with introductory gemstone material. The remainder of the book discusses, in chakra by chakra format, specific gemstones for healing work, their properties and uses.

0-87542-759-6, 336 pgs., 6 x 9, color plates, softcover   **$12.95**

DOWSING FOR HEALTH: The Applications & Methods for Holistic Healing
by Arthur Bailey

Now you can determine what your own body requires for wellness through the use of proven techniques from an experienced dowser. Learn how to detect food allergies, vitamin deficiencies and alternative remedies with the aid of a simple pendulum. The ability to dowse is not a gift that belongs to a chosen few; it is, in fact, present in everyone. *Dowsing for Health* explains exactly how to use this invaluable method to improve your own health and that of others.

0-87542-059-1, 176 pgs., 6 x 9, illus., softcover   **$9.95**

AWAKENING THE LIFE FORCE
The Philosophy & Psychology of "Spontaneous Yoga"
by Rajarshi Muni

This book is about higher yoga—not physical exercises or meditation to achieve inner peace and happiness (though these may be its by-products or used in preparation for higher yoga). *Awakening the Life Force* is about a proven process by which you can achieve, eternally, liberation from the limitations of time and space, unlimited divine powers, and an immortal, physically perfect divine body that is retained forever. The sages who composed the ancient scriptures achieved such a state, as have men and women of all religious traditions. How? Through the process of "spontaneous" yoga.

In spontaneous yoga, the body and mind are surrendered to the spontaneous workings of the awakened life force: prana. This awakened prana works in its own amazing way to purify the physical and nonphysical bodies of an individual. Whatever path, religion or teaching you follow, *Awakening the Life Force* can help you understand the fascinating physical and metaphysical cosmos in which you live. It reveals how anyone with genuine sincerity can practice dharma, or pure conscious living, which results in prosperity, pleasure, happiness, and the joy of selflessness.

0-87542-581-X, 224 pgs., 7 x 10, color plates, softcover $15.00

ENERGIZE!
The Alchemy of Breath & Movement for Health & Transformation
by Elrond, Juliana and Sophia Blawyn and Suzanne Jones

Meeting the needs of our daily obligations can drain us, frustrate us, and slowly kill us in both body and spirit. If you wish to pursue spiritual growth and you lack the strength to devote to this goal, this book can help. With just a few minutes a day of dynamic movement and consciously controlled breathing, you will begin to move your Chi, or vital energy, and you will experience heightened levels of physical energy, greater mental clarity, and a more fit and flexible body. As your reservoir of energy increases, your joy in life will increase, you will possess a greater capacity to function happily and productively in your daily life, and your spiritual progress begins.

Energize! blends the esoteric traditions of yoga, sufism and taoism. You have the remarkable opportunity to learn Chinese *T'ai Chi Chi Kung, T'ai Chi Ruler,* and Red Dragon *Chi Kung*; East Indian Chakra Energizers; Middle Eastern Sufi Earth Dancing, Veil Dancing and Whirling; and the Native American Dance of the Four Directions, all at your own pace in the privacy of your own home.

0-87542-060-5, 240 pgs., 6 x 9, 96 illus., softcover $10.00

THE HEALER'S MANUAL
A Beginner's Guide to Vibrational Therapies
Ted Andrews

Did you know that a certain Mozart symphony can ease digestion problems … that swelling often indicates being stuck in outworn patterns … that breathing pink is good for skin conditions and loneliness? Most dis-ease stems from a meta-physical base. While we are constantly being exposed to viruses and bacteria, it is our unbalanced or blocked emotions, attitudes and thoughts that deplete our natural physical energies and make us more susceptible to "catching a cold" or manifesting some other physical problem.

Healing, as approached in *The Healer's Manual,* involves locating and removing energy blockages wherever they occur—physical or otherwise. This book is an easy guide to simple vibrational healing therapies that anyone can learn to apply to restore homeostasis to their body's energy system. By employing sound, color, fragrance, etheric touch and flower/gem elixers, you can partici-pate actively within the healing of your body and the opening of higher percep-tions. You will discover that you can heal more aspects of your life than you ever thought possible.

0-87542-007-9, 256 pgs., 6 x 9, illus., softcover $10.00

HOW TO HEAL WITH COLOR
by Ted Andrews

Now, for perhaps the first time, color therapy is placed within the grasp of the average individual. Anyone can learn to facilitate and accelerate the healing process on all levels with the simple color therapies in *How to Heal with Color*.

Color serves as a vibrational remedy that interacts with the human energy sys-tem to stabilize physical, emotional, mental and spiritual conditions. When there is balance, we can more effectively rid ourselves of toxins, negativities and pat-terns that hinder our life processes.

This book provides color application guidelines that are beneficial for over 50 physical conditions and a wide variety of emotional and mental conditions. Receive simple and tangible instructions for performing "muscle testing" on yourself and others to find the most beneficial colors. Learn how to apply color therapy through touch, projection, breathing, cloth, water and candles. Learn how to use the little known but powerful color-healing system of the mystical Qabala to balance and open the psychic centers. Plus, discover simple techniques for performing long distance healings on others.

0-87542-005-2, 240 pgs., mass market, illus. $3.95

MEDITATION & HUMAN GROWTH
A Practical Manual for Higher Consciousness
by Genevieve Lewis Paulson

Meditation has many purposes—healing, past life awareness, balance, mental clarity and relaxation are just a few. *Meditation and Human Growth* is a life-long guidebook that focuses on the practice of meditation as a tool for growth and development, as well as for expanding consciousness into other realms. It includes detailed meditations of both a "practical" and more esoteric nature to serve the needs of the complete person. Specific exercises are provided for different areas of life: health of the physical body; wealth in the physical world; emotional well-being; transmuting excess sexual energy; experiencing oneness with the universe; and alignment with the seasonal, lunar and planetary energies.

Meditation is a way of opening into areas that are beyond our normal thinking patterns. In fact, what we now call "altered states" and "peak experiences" will become the normal consciousness of the future. This book is full of techniques for those who wish to claim those higher vibrations and expanded awareness for their lives today.

ISBN: 0-87542-599-2, est. 256 pgs., 17 illus., 4 color plates, $12.95

PERSONAL ALCHEMY
A Handbook of Healing & Self-Transformation
by Amber Wolfe

Personal Alchemy offers the first bold look at the practical use of "Rays" for healing and self-development. Rays are spontaneous energy emanations emitting a specific quality, property or attribute. The Red Ray, for example, represents the energies of life force, survival and strength. When used in conjunction with active imagery, the alchemical properties of the Red Ray can activate independence, release inferiority, or realign destructiveness and frustration. *Personal Alchemy* explains each color Ray and Light in depth, in a manner designed to teach the material and to encourage the active participation of the reader.

What's more, this book goes beyond anything else written on the Rays because it contains an extensive set of alchemical correlations that amplify the Ray's powers. Each Ray correlates with a specific element, harmonic sound, aroma, symbol, person, rune, astrological sign, Tarot card, angel, and stone, so there are numerous ways to experience and learn this system of healing magick.

0-87542-890-8, 592 pgs., 7 x 10, illus., softcover $17.95